Respiratory Emergencies

Editors

ROBERT J. VISSERS
MICHAEL A. GIBBS

EMERGENCY MEDICINE
CLINICS OF NORTH AMERICA

www.emed.theclinics.com

Consulting Editor
AMAL MATTU

February 2016 • Volume 34 • Number 1

ELSEVIER

1600 John F. Kennedy Boulevard • Suite 1800 • Philadelphia, Pennsylvania, 19103-2899

http://www.theclinics.com

EMERGENCY MEDICINE CLINICS OF NORTH AMERICA Volume 34, Number 1
February 2016 ISSN 0733-8627, ISBN-13: 978-0-323-41328-2

Editor: Patrick Manley
Developmental Editor: Casey Jackson

Emergency Medicine Clinics of North America (ISSN 0733-8627) is published quarterly by Elsevier Inc., 360 Park Avenue South, New York, NY, 10010-1710. Months of issue are February, May, August, and November. Business and Editorial Offices: 1600 John F. Kennedy Boulevard, Suite 1800, Philadelphia, PA 19103-2899. Customer Service Office: 6277 Sea Harbor Drive, Orlando, FL 32887-4800. Periodicals postage paid at New York, NY, and additional mailing offices. Subscription prices are $100.00 per year (US students), $320.00 per year (US individuals), $579.00 per year (US institutions), $220.00 per year (international students), $450.00 per year (international individuals), $711.00 per year (international institutions), $220.00 per year (Canadian students), $385.00 per year (Canadian individuals), and $711.00 per year (Canadian institutions). International air speed delivery is included in all *Clinics'* subscription prices. All prices are subject to change without notice. **POSTMASTER:** Send address changes to *Emergency Medicine Clinics of North America*, Elsevier Periodicals Customer Service, 11830 Westline Industrial Drive, St. Louis, MO 63146. Customer Service (orders, claims, online, change of address): Elsevier Periodicals **Customer Service, 11830 Westline Industrial Drive, St. Louis, MO 63146. Tel: 1-800-654-2452 (U.S. and Canada); 314-453-7041 (outside U.S. and Canada). Fax: 314-453-5170. E-mail: journalscustomerservice-usa@elsevier.com (for print support);** journalsonlinesupport-usa@elsevier.com (for online support).

Reprints. For copies of 100 or more of articles in this publication, please contact the Commercial Reprints Department, Elsevier Inc., 360 Park Avenue South, New York, NY 10010-1710. Tel.: 212-633-3874; Fax: 212-633-3820; E-mail: reprints@elsevier.com.

Emergency Medicine Clinics of North America is covered in *MEDLINE/PubMed (Index Medicus), Current Contents/Clinical Medicine, EMBASE/Excerpta Medica, BIOSIS, SciSearch, CINAHL, ISI/BIOMED,* and *Research Alert.*

Contributors

CONSULTING EDITOR

AMAL MATTU, MD, FAAEM, FACEP
Professor and Vice Chair, Department of Emergency Medicine, University of Maryland School of Medicine, Baltimore, Maryland

EDITORS

ROBERT J. VISSERS, MD, MBA
President and CEO, Boulder Community Health, Boulder, Colorado; Adjunct Associate Professor Emergency Medicine, Oregon Health Sciences University, Portland, Oregon

MICHAEL A. GIBBS, MD
Professor and Chairman, Department of Emergency Medicine, Carolinas Medical Center, Charlotte, North Carolina

AUTHORS

MICHAEL G. ALLISON, MD
Attending Physician, Critical Care Medicine, St. Agnes Hospital, Baltimore, Maryland

JUSTIN O. COOK, MD, FACEP
Emergency Physician, Northwest Acute Care Specialists, Portland, Oregon

PETER M.C. DeBLIEUX, MD, FAAEM
Professor of Emergency Medicine and Critical Care, Louisiana State University, University Medical Center of New Orleans, New Orleans, Louisiana

ELIZABETH DEVOS, MD, MPH, FACEP
Assistant Professor, Department of Emergency Medicine, University of Florida College of Medicine - Jacksonville, Jacksonville, Florida

ALAN C. HEFFNER, MD
Division of Critical Care Medicine, Department of Internal Medicine, Carolinas Medical Center; Director, Medical ICU, Director of ECMO Services Pulmonary and Critical Care Consultants, Department of Emergency Medicine, Carolinas Medical Center, University of North Carolina, Charlotte Campus, Charlotte, North Carolina

ZARETH IRWIN, MD, FACEP
Emergency Physician, Northwest Acute Care Specialists, Portland, Oregon

LISA JACOBSON, MD, FACEP
Assistant Professor, Department of Emergency Medicine, University of Florida College of Medicine - Jacksonville, Jacksonville, Florida

HANEY MALLEMAT, MD
Assistant Professor of Emergency Medicine, University of Maryland School of Medicine, Baltimore, Maryland

MICHAEL C. OVERBECK, MD
Assistant Professor, Department of Emergency Medicine, University of Colorado School of Medicine, Aurora, Colorado

THOMAS M. PRZYBYSZ, MD
Division of Critical Care Medicine, Department of Internal Medicine, Carolinas Medical Center, Charlotte, North Carolina

AMBER M. RICHARDS, MD
Department of Emergency Medicine, Maine Medical Center, Assistant Professor, Tufts University School of Medicine, Portland, Maine

RORY SPIEGEL, MD
Clinical Instructor, Department of Emergency Medicine, Stony Brook Medical Center, Stony Brook, New York

DANE STEVENSON, MD
Geriatric Emergency Medicine Fellow, Department of Emergency Medicine, University of California, Davis, Sacramento, California

SALVADOR J. SUAU, MD, FAAEM
Assistant Professor of Emergency Medicine, Louisiana State University, University Medical Center of New Orleans, New Orleans, Louisiana

KATREN TYLER, MD
Associate Professor, Associate Program Director, Geriatric Emergency Medicine Fellowship Director, Vice Chair for Faculty Development, Wellness and Outreach, Department of Emergency Medicine, University of California, Davis, Sacramento, California

MICHAEL E. WINTERS, MD, FACEP, FAAEM
Associate Professor of Emergency Medicine and Medicine, Co-Director, Emergency Medicine/Internal Medicine/Critical Care Program, University of Maryland School of Medicine, Baltimore, Maryland

Contents

Acute respiratory distress syndrome (ARDS) is defined by acute diffuse inflammatory lung injury invoked by a variety of systemic or pulmonary insults. Despite medical progress in management, mortality remains 27% to 45%. Patients with ARDS should be managed with low tidal volume ventilation. Permissive hypercapnea is well tolerated. Conservative fluid strategy can reduce ventilator and hospital days in patients without shock. Prone positioning and neuromuscular blockers reduce mortality in some patients. Early management of ARDS is relevant to emergency medicine. Identifying ARDS patients who should be transferred to an extracorporeal membrane oxygenation center is an important task for emergency providers.

Acute asthma and chronic obstructive pulmonary disease (COPD) exacerbations are the most common respiratory diseases requiring emergent medical evaluation and treatment. Asthma and COPD are chronic, debilitating disease processes that have been differentiated traditionally by the presence or absence of reversible airflow obstruction. Asthma and COPD exacerbations impose an enormous economic burden on the US health care budget. In daily clinical practice, it is difficult to differentiate these 2 obstructive processes based on their symptoms, and on their nearly identical acute treatment strategies, major differences are important when discussing anatomic sites involved, long-term prognosis, and the nature of inflammatory markers.

Acute dyspnea in older patients is a common presentation to the emergency department. Acute dyspnea in older adults is often the consequence of multiple overlapping disorders, such as pneumonia precipitating acute heart failure. Emergency physicians must be comfortable managing patients with acute dyspnea of uncertain cause and varying goals of care. In addition to the important role noninvasive ventilation (NIV) plays in full resuscitation, NIV can be useful as a method of providing supportive or nearly fully supportive care while more information is gathered from the patients and their loved ones.

Noninvasive ventilation (NIV) improves oxygenation and ventilation, prevents endotracheal intubation, and decreases the mortality rate in select patients with acute respiratory failure. Although NIV is used commonly for acute exacerbations of chronic obstructive pulmonary disease and acute cardiogenic pulmonary edema, there are emerging indications for its use in the emergency department. Emergency physicians must be knowledgeable regarding the indications and contraindications for NIV in emergency department patients with acute respiratory failure as well as the means of initiating it and monitoring patients who are receiving it.

Mechanical ventilation has a long and storied history, but until recently the process required little from the emergency physician. In the modern emergency department, critically ill patients spend a longer period under the care of the emergency physician, requiring a greater understanding of ventilator management. This article serves as an introduction to mechanical ventilation and a user-friendly bedside guide.

Respiratory emergencies are one of the most common reasons parents seek evaluation for the their children in the emergency department (ED) each year, and respiratory failure is the most common cause of cardiopulmonary arrest in pediatric patients. Whereas many respiratory illnesses are mild and self-limiting, others are life threatening and require prompt diagnosis and management. Therefore, it is imperative that emergency clinicians be able to promptly recognize and manage these illnesses. This article reviews ED diagnosis and management of foreign body aspiration, asthma exacerbation, epiglottitis, bronchiolitis, community-acquired pneumonia, and pertussis.

 Video showing Demonstration of the reduction in anatomic deadspace with high flow nasal oxygen accompanies this article

Patients in respiratory distress often require airway management, including endotracheal intubation. It takes a methodical approach to transition from an unstable patient in distress with an unsecured airway, to a stable, sedated patient with a definitive airway. Through a deliberate course of advanced preparation, the emergency physician can tailor the approach to the individual clinical situation and optimize the chance of first-pass success. Sedation of the intubated patient confers physiologic benefits and should be included in the plan for airway control.

Elizabeth DeVos and Lisa Jacobson

Undifferentiated patients in respiratory distress require immediate attention in the emergency department. Using a thorough history and clinical examination, clinicians can determine the most likely causes of dyspnea. Understanding the pathophysiology of the most common diseases contributing to dyspnea guides rational testing and informed, expedited treatment decisions.

Zareth Irwin and Justin O. Cook

 Videos of various normal and abnormal lung ultrasound findings accompany this article

Pulmonary ultrasound continues to develop and is ideally suited for the evaluation and treatment of respiratory emergencies. It is portable, can be performed rapidly, has no ionizing radiation, and is highly sensitive and specific for the diagnosis of pneumothorax, pneumonia, pulmonary edema, and free fluid in the chest.

EMERGENCY MEDICINE
CLINICS OF NORTH AMERICA

PROGRAM OBJECTIVE

The goal of *Emergency Medicine Clinics of North America* is to keep practicing emergency medicine physicians and emergency medicine residents up to date with current clinical practice in emergency medicine by providing timely articles reviewing the state of the art in patient care.

LEARNING OBJECTIVES

Upon completion of this activity, participants will be able to:

1. Review management strategies for respiratory emergencies in special populations, such as geriatric and pediatric populations.
2. Recognize and discuss the use of mechanical and non-invasive ventilation in emergency situations.
3. Discuss techniques in airway management to optimize patient outcome in respiratory failure.

ACCREDITATION

The Elsevier Office of Continuing Medical Education (EOCME) is accredited by the Accreditation Council for Continuing Medical Education (ACCME) to provide continuing medical education for physicians.

The EOCME designates this enduring material for a maximum of 15 *AMA PRA Category 1 Credit*(s)™. Physicians should claim only the credit commensurate with the extent of their participation in the activity.

All other health care professionals requesting continuing education credit for this enduring material will be issued a certificate of participation.

DISCLOSURE OF CONFLICTS OF INTEREST

The EOCME assesses conflict of interest with its instructors, faculty, planners, and other individuals who are in a position to control the content of CME activities. All relevant conflicts of interest that are identified are thoroughly vetted by EOCME for fair balance, scientific objectivity, and patient care recommendations. EOCME is committed to providing its learners with CME activities that promote improvements or quality in healthcare and not a specific proprietary business or a commercial interest.

The planning committee, staff, authors and editors listed below have identified no financial relationships or relationships to products or devices they or their spouse/life partner have with commercial interest related to the content of this CME activity:

Michael G. Allison, MD; Justin O. Cook, MD, FACEP; Peter M.C. DeBlieux, MD, FAAEM; Elizabeth DeVos, MD, MPH, FACEP; Anjali Fortna; Michael A. Gibbs, MD; Alan C. Heffner, MD; Zareth Irwin, MD, FACEP; Lisa Jacobson, MD, FACEP; Indu Kumari; Haney Mallemat, MD; Patrick Manley; Amal Mattu, MD, FAAEM, FACEP; Michael C. Overbeck, MD; Thomas M. Przybysz, MD; Amber M. Richards, MD; Rory Spiegel, MD; Dane Stevenson, MD; Salvador J. Suau, MD, FAAEM; Erin Scheckenbach; Katren Tyler, MD; Robert J. Vissers, MD, MBA; Michael E. Winters, MD, FACEP, FAAEM.

UNAPPROVED/OFF-LABEL USE DISCLOSURE

The EOCME requires CME faculty to disclose to the participants:

1. When products or procedures being discussed are off-label, unlabelled, experimental, and/or investigational (not US Food and Drug Administration [FDA] approved); and
2. Any limitations on the information presented, such as data that are preliminary or that represent ongoing research, interim analyses, and/or unsupported opinions. Faculty may discuss information about pharmaceutical agents that is outside of FDA-approved labelling. This information is intended solely for CME and is not intended to promote off-label use of these medications. If you have any questions, contact the medical affairs department of the manufacturer for the most recent prescribing information.

TO ENROLL

To enroll in the *Emergency Medicine Clinics* Continuing Medical Education program, call customer service at 1-800-654-2452 or sign up online at http://www.theclinics.com/home/cme. The CME program is available to subscribers for an additional annual fee of $235 USD.

METHOD OF PARTICIPATION

In order to claim credit, participants must complete the following:

1. Complete enrolment as indicated above.

2. Read the activity.
3. Complete the CME Test and Evaluation. Participants must achieve a score of 70% on the test. All CME Tests and Evaluations must be completed online.

CME INQUIRIES/SPECIAL NEEDS
For all CME inquiries or special needs, please contact elsevierCME@elsevier.com.

Foreword

Pulmonary Emergencies

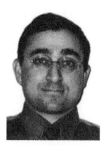

Amal Mattu, MD, FAAEM, FACEP
Consulting Editor

The priority in acute resuscitation in emergency medicine is focused on the traditional mantra of "A-B-C"—airway, breath sounds, and circulation. The first two components of this mantra focus on the pulmonary system. Loss of airway function and compromise of lung function are the most rapid killers in emergency medicine, so it's appropriate that they receive the first and foremost attention in acute resuscitation. It is also appropriate, therefore, that airway training and understanding of pulmonary function are critical for competency in our specialty. Quite simply, if a provider possesses clinical excellence with the "A" and the "B," then lives are saved. Conversely, if a provider lacks skills in the "A" and the "B," then patients die...very quickly.

In this issue of *Emergency Medicine Clinics of North America*, Drs Robert Vissers and Michael Gibbs have assembled a group of authors to write a tutorial on how to manage the "A" and "B" with clinical excellence. Drs Vissers and Gibbs, both of whom are national experts in critical care and airway management, in particular focus the readers' attention on the most common and the most deadly of pulmonary emergencies. The editors and authors address bread-and-butter emergency conditions, such as the approach to dyspnea and exacerbations of chronic obstructive pulmonary disease and asthma. They also address acute respiratory distress syndrome. Special populations, such as pediatrics and geriatrics, are addressed. Noninvasive and invasive forms of mechanical ventilation are discussed. Finally, the cutting-edge topic of lung ultrasound is described for the diagnosis of the various pulmonary diseases.

In total, this issue of *Emergency Medicine Clinics of North America* is an important contribution to the reading curriculum of every practicing emergency care provider. The pearls and pitfalls discussed within this issue are certain to improve everyone's practice and to help save lives. Following a study of this issue of *Emergency Medicine*

Emerg Med Clin N Am 34 (2016) xi–xii
http://dx.doi.org/10.1016/j.emc.2015.10.003
0733-8627/16/$ – see front matter © 2016 Published by Elsevier Inc.

Clinics of North America, every reader is certain to gain a greater level of knowledge and competence in dealing with emergencies of the "A" and the "B."

Amal Mattu, MD, FAAEM, FACEP
Department of Emergency Medicine
University of Maryland School of Medicine
Baltimore, MD 21201, USA

E-mail address:
amalmattu@comcast.net

Preface

Respiratory Emergencies

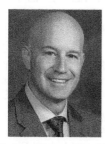 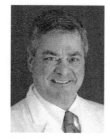

Robert J. Vissers, MD, MBA   Michael A. Gibbs, MD
Editors

For breath is life, so if you breathe well you will live long on earth.
—Sanskrit Proverb

Our ability to breathe…so fundamental that we not dare imagine ever depriving ourselves of this basic function, even for a brief moment. It therefore follows that acute respiratory emergencies are both terrifying to the patient and challenging to even the most seasoned clinician. Simply stated, the stakes are high for both the patient and the physician. With this challenge comes equal reward when a skilled Emergency Department team, acting swiftly and with sophistication, is able to convert a young dying asthmatic, or a patient with acute decompensated chronic obstructive pulmonary disease, into someone recovered, and finally able to muster a tentative smile… breathing restored.

For the emergency clinician managing the acutely dyspneic patient, several important serial action steps must be taken:

First: A rapid assessment of acute dyspnea must yield the correct working diagnosis or diagnoses.

Second: Once a working diagnosis has been established, targeted therapy must proceed aggressively and without delay.

Third: The patient must be continuously and frequently reassessed to ensure that the response to therapy is appropriate, and the care team must be ready to quickly change course if progress is not being made.

In the pages that follow, this issue of the *Emergency Medicine Clinics of North America* approaches this complex topic by: (1) discussing the assessment and management of acute respiratory distress in adults, children, and geriatric patients; (2) summarizing the cutting-edge use of point-of-care ultrasound in acute dyspnea; (3) outlining state-of-the-art airway and ventilator management, and noninvasive ventilation techniques;

Emerg Med Clin N Am 34 (2016) xiii–xiv
http://dx.doi.org/10.1016/j.emc.2015.10.002
0733-8627/16/$ – see front matter © 2016 Published by Elsevier Inc.

emed.theclinics.com

and (4) describing an evidence-based approach to the emergency care of acute asthma, COPD, and ARDS.

Restating the challenge that lies in front of us…high risk, high reward.

Robert J. Vissers, MD, MBA
President and CEO
Boulder Community Health
Boulder, CO, USA

Adjunct Associate Professor Emergency Medicine
Oregon Health Sciences University
Portland, OR, USA

Michael A. Gibbs, MD
Department of Emergency Medicine
Carolinas Medical Center
Charlotte, NC 28203, USA

E-mail addresses:
rvissers1@me.com (R.J. Vissers)
Michael.Gibbs@carolinashealthcare.org (M.A. Gibbs)

Erratum

Errors were made in the November 2015 issue (Volume 33, Number 4) of *Emergency Medicine Clinics*. On page 779 of the article "New Drugs of Abuse and Withdrawal Syndromes," the third author's name should read: "Nidal Moukaddam, MD, PhD." On page 825 of the article "Psychiatric Emergencies in the Elderly" the third author's name should read "Sagar Galwankar, DNB, MPH, Diplomat. ABEM" and the affiliations for this author are as follows: "Department of Emergency Medicine, University of Florida, Jacksonville, FL, USA."

http://dx.doi.org/10.1016/j.emc.2015.11.001
0733-8627/16/$ – see front matter Published by Elsevier Inc.
emed.theclinics.com

Early Treatment of Severe Acute Respiratory Distress Syndrome

Thomas M. Przybysz, MD[a], Alan C. Heffner, MD[a,b],*

KEYWORDS

- Acute respiratory distress syndrome • Acute respiratory failure • Hypoxia
- Hypoxemia • Severe ARDS

KEY POINTS

- Severe acute respiratory distress syndrome (ARDS) is a life-threatening condition characterized by acute bilateral pulmonary infiltrates occurring after a recognizable trigger and a Pao_2 to fraction of inspired oxygen (Fio_2) ratio of less than 100.
- Patients with all severities of ARDS should be managed with a low tidal volume strategy, safe plateau pressures, and fluid restriction as tolerated by hemodynamics.
- Patients with severe ARDS should receive early neuromuscular blockade and consideration for prone ventilation. Patients with severe ARDS not responding to therapy should be transferred to an ECMO center.

INTRODUCTION

ARDS is a rare but life-threatening syndrome characterized by acute bilateral inflammatory pulmonary infiltrates and severe hypoxia. US cases were estimated at 86 per 100,000 individuals, with 74,500 annual deaths in 2005.[1–3] ARDS survival has improved due to advances in supportive care but mortality remains at 27% to 45% depending on the severity of ARDS. ARDS is classified into physiologic and prognostic categories of mild, moderate, and severe based on Pao_2 to Fio_2 (P/F) ratio (200–300, 100–200, and <100, respectively).[4]

ARDS may be triggered by pulmonary and nonpulmonary insults. It most commonly occurs in patients with acute critical illness due to sepsis, pneumonia, and trauma,

[a] Division of Critical Care Medicine, Department of Internal Medicine, Carolinas Medical Center, 1000 Blyth Boulevard, Charlotte, NC 28203, USA; [b] Medical ICU, Department of Emergency Medicine, Carolinas Medical Center, University of North Carolina, Charlotte Campus, 1000 Blyth Boulevard, Charlotte, NC 28203, USA
* Corresponding author. Medical ICU, Department of Emergency Medicine, Carolinas Medical Center, University of North Carolina, Charlotte Campus, 1000 Blyth Boulevard, Charlotte, NC 28203.
E-mail address: Alan.heffner@carolinashealthcare.org

Emerg Med Clin N Am 34 (2016) 1–14
http://dx.doi.org/10.1016/j.emc.2015.08.001
0733-8627/16/$ – see front matter © 2016 Elsevier Inc. All rights reserved.

where it is often accompanied by multiorgan dysfunction. Primary lung disease may be the initial or sole manifestation of acute severe ARDS in some cases, with pulmonary aspiration and near-drowning 2 common examples. This review discusses the clinical presentation of ARDS and provides an evidence-based approach to the early management of ARDS pertinent to emergency medicine physicians, with a focus on severe ARDS.

CLINICAL PRESENTATION AND ACUTE RESPIRATORY DISTRESS SYNDROME DEFINITION

Patients with ARDS exhibit hypoxemia associated with acute bilateral pulmonary infiltrates occurring within 1 week of a provoking insult. Intubation and mechanical ventilation with a high F_{IO_2} are often required to compensate for the large alveolar-arterial oxygen gradient. The former definition of ARDS and acute lung injury required exclusion of left atrial hypertension causing hydrostatic pulmonary edema. The revised criteria, however, removed this strict criteria, recognizing that inflammatory lung disease and elevated left atrial pressures are not mutually exclusive.[4]

The pathophysiology of ARDS includes increased pulmonary vascular permeability, loss of aerated lung, decreased lung compliance, and increase in physiologic dead space. The damaged capillaries allow protein-rich fluid to overwhelm the normal lymphatic drainage of the lung.[5] Chest radiograph (CXR) frequently demonstrates diffuse and homogeneous infiltrates; however, CT scans often reveal a heterogeneous pattern of dependent consolidation.[6]

PATIENT EVALUATION

Hypoxia with acute bilateral infiltrates after a known trigger associated with ARDS is clinically diagnostic (**Table 1**). Usually a diagnosis of ARDS is determined with a good patient history, physical examination, and CXR data. Some patients develop ARDS during an emergency room course (eg, worsening sepsis, aspiration, and influenza), which can be overlooked without a high index of suspicion. Occasionally patients with ARDS present without a known trigger or an incomplete history, which makes a diagnosis of ARDS more difficult to confirm. Incomplete patient history and nonspecific time-consuming diagnostics are early hurdles in quickly identifying the inciting cause of ARDS for some atypical presentations and other causes for bilateral infiltrates should be considered (**Table 2**). Hydrostatic pulmonary edema commonly mimics ARDS and can be difficult to correctly identify. CXRs have limited

Table 1 Conditions associated with acute respiratory distress syndrome	
Sepsis	Pulmonary contusion
Aspiration	After upper airway obstruction
Infectious pneumonia	Stem cell transplant
Trauma	Drug reaction
Burn	Venous air embolism
Blood product transfusion	Amniotic fluid embolism
Cardiopulmonary bypass	Neurogenic pulmonary edema
Pancreatitis	Acute eosinophilic pneumonia
Drug overdose	Bronchiolitis obliterans organizing pneumonia
Near drowning	Smoke inhalation

Table 2
Mimics of acute respiratory distress syndrome

Disease	Test	Comment
Pulmonary edema	BNP	Not specific for heart failure
	CXR	Unable to distinguish reliably from ARDS
	Chest CT	Useful at distinguishing from ARDS
	Echocardiogram	Not sensitive for diastolic dysfunction or volume overload. ARDS can cause stress-induced systolic dysfunction
	Lung ultrasound	Promising but needs to be verified in larger study
Atelectasis	None	Should improve with proper recruitment
Diffuse alveolar hemorrhage	Bronchoscopy or biopsy	Treat underlying disease
Eosinophilic pneumonia	Bronchoscopy or biopsy	May respond to steroids
Malignancy	Biopsy	Treat underlying disease
Hypersensitivity pneumonitis	Exposure history, bronchoscopy, and biopsy	Remove inciting antigen

value in distinguishing these 2 types of edema as do laboratory tests.[7] Brain natriuretic peptide (BNP) values can be elevated in both ARDS and heart failure.[8,9] BNP less than 100 pg/mL, however, makes heart failure an unlikely cause of bilateral pulmonary infiltrates.[10] Echocardiography is useful to evaluate factors associated with elevated left atrial pressure, such as systolic dysfunction and valvular disease, but is less accurate in evaluating diastolic dysfunction. Although the morphology of pulmonary infiltrates on CT is more useful in differentiating hydrostatic edema from inflammatory ARDS, obtaining CT imaging may not be feasible in an unstable patient.[11] It is also important to remember that patients do not always follow classic clinical categories. As an example, ARDS triggers may also provoke stress-induced cardiomyopathy, making pure clinical differentiation of inflammatory and hydrostatic edema difficult.[12]

Bedside lung ultrasound is a helpful diagnostic tool. A small study of pulmonary edema patients suggests clinical utility of bedside lung ultrasound in distinguishing inflammatory and hydrostatic edema.[13] Different ultrasound images for ARDS and hydrostatic edema are seen in **Figs. 1** and **2**. Spared areas, pleural abnormalities, and consolidation favor inflammatory infiltrates, whereas large effusions, smooth thin pleural line, and diffuse homogenous alveolar-interstitial syndrome (or white lung) suggest hydrostatic edema (**Table 3**). Although this study needs to be confirmed in a larger cohort, the results are encouraging and may allow for improved accuracy and rapid bedside diagnosis of severe ARDS.

Diffuse alveolar hemorrhage, eosinophilic pneumonia, hypersensitivity pneumonitis, and malignancy can also present similarly to ARDS. Bronchoscopy and open lung biopsy are generally required to confirm these diagnoses.

EARLY MANAGEMENT

The main priorities of early ARDS management are maintenance of systemic oxygen delivery (DO_2) and avoidance of iatrogenic ventilator-induced lung injury. Always

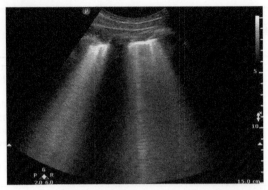

Fig. 1. Lung ultrasound of patient with ARDS. Note the pleural abnormalities. (*Courtesy of* Jacob Avila.)

remember, the physiologic goals in ARDS management are not intuitive. Strict therapeutic normalization of pH, Pco_2, and Po_2 is associated with adverse outcomes, as evidenced by the 9% absolute mortality increase in the ARDSNet trial control group, despite higher arterial oxygen saturation (SaO_2) levels during the first 24 hours of care.[14] Similarly, permissive hypercapnea, which prioritizes safe low tidal volume mechanical ventilation at the expense of systemic hypercapnea, is associated with improved outcomes.[15,16]

SaO_2 is easily measured, but the ideal target in ARDS is unknown and may be difficult to standardize because systemic DO_2 is the more important variable correlating with ARDS patient survival.[17,18] The relationship between DO_2 and SaO_2 is described in Equation 1. Despite poor oxygenation and impaired DO_2, a majority of ARDS deaths are attributed to multiorgan failure rather than refractory hypoxemia.[19]

$$DO_2 = [1.39 \times Hgb \times SaO_2 + (0.003 \times Pao_2)] \times \text{cardiac output} \tag{1}$$

Cardiac output (CO) has a linear relationship to systemic DO_2 and many patients have physiologic reserve to dramatically augment CO in the context of severe critical illness. Adequacy of SaO_2 in severe lung disease requires interpretation in the context

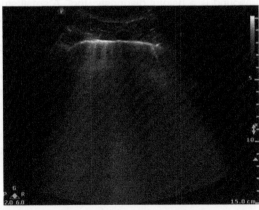

Fig. 2. Lung ultrasound of a patient with hydrostatic edema. Note the thin smooth pleural line. (*Courtesy of* Jacob Avila.)

Table 3
Differentiation of acute respiratory distress syndrome and pulmonary edema with lung ultrasound

Characteristics of Acute Respiratory Distress Syndrome	Characteristics of Pulmonary Edema
Alveolar-interstitial syndrome	Alveolar-interstitial syndrome
Pleural line abnormality	Large pleural effusions
Reduction of lung sliding	Homogeneous pattern
Spared areas	—
Consolidation	—
Small pleural effusion	—

of systemic hemodynamics. Rather than focusing on the hemoglobin saturation, the early goals of care for severe ARDS patients are maintaining systemic DO_2, optimizing hemodynamics, and minimizing ongoing lung injury. Patients can die early from severe ARDS and it is important to have a strategy to deal with life-threatening hypoxia (**Table 4**).

TREATMENT OF LIFE-THREATENING HYPOXIA
Fraction of Inspired Oxygen

The quickest and simplest method of improving oxygenation is increasing FIO_2 delivery. Knowledge of the delivery systems designed to provide supplemental oxygen is important. For example, the term, *100% nonrebreather*, is a misnomer. Respiratory DO_2 depends on patient-specific respiratory mechanics, such as minute ventilation, inspiratory flow, and work of breathing. For a fixed nasal cannula flow rate, there is significant variability of delivered oxygen among healthy volunteers.[20] In the setting of high minute ventilation, the FIO_2 delivered to alveoli is simply diluted by entrainment of ambient air.[21]

Newer humidified high-flow nasal cannulas (**Fig. 3**) can deliver measured FIO_2 closer to machine-set FIO_2, provided the flow rates are high (30–60 liters per minute [lpm]), which allows these devices to provide higher FIO_2 than traditional face masks.[22] Although a majority of patients with ARDS ultimately require mechanical ventilation, understanding the limits of supplemental oxygen should improve patient safety (**Table 5**). ARDS patients are at increased risk for peri-intubation complications and

Table 4
Life-threatening hypoxia therapies

Physiologic Methods to Improve Life-Threatening Hypoxemia	
Increase FIO_2	Confirm delivery of 100% oxygen
Increase mean airway pressure	Optimize MAP while monitoring plateau pressure and CO
Recruit more alveoli	Perform RMs, clear secretions, increase PEEP, treat pneumothorax if present, prone positioning, check for dynamic hyperinflation
Improve lung diffusion	Assess for response to diuretics or need for ultrafiltration
Improve or redistribute blood flow	Assess CO and add inotropes if indicated, prone positioning, inhaled NO, inhaled epoprostenol
Add extracorporeal support	VV-ECMO, VA-ECMO

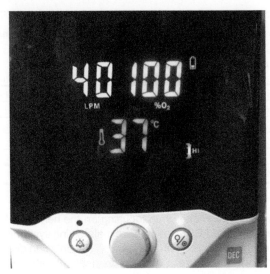

Fig. 3. Typical setup for a humidified high-flow nasal cannula in a patient with severe hypoxia.

death due to limited pulmonary reserve and hypoxia. Noninvasive ventilation and humidified high-flow nasal cannulas are capable of delivering higher FIO_2 than simple face masks, Venturi masks, and nonrebreathers; consequently, they are useful tools to preoxygenate prior to intubation.

Patients with severe ARDS are tenuous and the most skilled provider available should be in charge of safely securing their airways. Rapid sequence intubation with neuromuscular blocking agents is highly recommended given its association with reduced aspiration and death.[23] Safely intubating hypoxic patients is an important skill but is not discussed at length in this review. Information about preoxygenation and about reducing peri-intubation morbidity and mortality is found at www.emcrit.org and in the article on airway management elsewhere in this issue.

Mean Airway Pressure

After optimizing FIO_2, the next maneuvers should focus on increasing mean airway pressure. Positive pressure ventilation associated with mechanical ventilation increases mean airway pressure and, thereby, recruits functional but collapsed lung. Increasing mean airway pressure also independently raises the partial pressure of

Table 5		
Supplemental oxygen devices and delivered fraction of inspired oxygen		
	Flow	**Delivered Fraction of Inspired Oxygen**
Nasal cannula	1–6 lpm	24%–40%
Simple mask	5–10 lpm	35%–50%
Partial or nonrebreather	15 lpm	40%–80%
Humidified high-flow cannula	30–60 lpm	Near the set FIO_2 (21%–100%)
Noninvasive ventilation	Closed system	Set FIO_2
Mechanical ventilation	Closed system	Set FIO_2

alveolar oxygen in the alveoli (P_{AO_2}) and, consequently, the Pa_{O_2}, based on the alveolar gas equation:

$$P_{AO_2} = F_{IO_2} (P_{atm} - pH_2O) - (Pa_{CO_2}/RQ)$$

During positive pressure ventilation, mean airway pressure is added to atmospheric pressure (P_{atm}) in the alveolar gas equation. This additional increase in P_{AO_2} becomes significant in patients requiring high mean airway pressures associated with severe ARDS.[24]

Most ventilators calculate mean airway pressure as the average pressure applied during a respiratory cycle. Mean airway pressure is dependent on the area under the pressure-time curve. Increasing the area under this curve via positive end-expiratory pressure (PEEP), respiratory rate, tidal volume, and inspiratory time all generate higher mean airway pressures. Higher mean airway pressures tend to improve oxygenation and lead to lower F_{IO_2} requirements, although the clinical benefit of improved SaO_2 does not translate to improved survival among most ARDS patients. Despite improvements in lung function, reduced organ failure days, and reduced need for pulmonary rescue therapies, high-quality studies on high PEEP levels versus low PEEP levels failed to show a mortality benefit.[25,26] A 2010 meta-analysis showed an association between high PEEP levels and decreased mortality in moderate to severe ARDS (P/F ratio <200) but possible harm in patients with P/F ratio 200 to 300, suggesting higher PEEP levels should be avoided in mild ARDS.[27]

Reanalysis of 4 ARDS studies also reveals that driving pressure (plateau pressure minus PEEP, often referred to as deltaP) is strongly associated with mortality.[28] This suggests patient-specific factors and lung mechanics may aid in determining which patients benefit from higher levels of PEEP. This study found an association with the protective effects of higher PEEP levels only if they led to improved lung compliance. As such, PEEP levels higher than those routinely used in the ARDSNet PEEP-F_{IO_2} tables may be beneficial only when associated with improved lung compliance.

A seemingly more physiologic strategy at optimizing PEEP is guided by esophageal pressure measurements.[29] A recent study recruited 61 patients with ARDS and randomized them to either standard care with PEEP based on a PEEP to F_{IO_2} table or PEEP based on transpulmonary pressure (estimated to be PEEP minus esophageal pressure at end expiration). The goal transpulmonary pressure in this study at end-expiration was 0 cm H_2O to 10 cm H_2O based on severity of hypoxia, with 10 cm H_2O if the F_{IO_2} required was 95% or higher. The esophageal-guided PEEP group had significantly increased P/F ratios (90 points better), improved compliance, higher average Pa_{O_2}, higher average PEEP levels, and higher average mean airway pressure. The study was not powered to evaluate mortality but there is a study currently recruiting patients (NCT01681225) by the same group. The primary outcome is a composite of death and time off the ventilator at 28 days.

Recruitment

The best way to recruit alveoli for a specific patient with ARDS depends on the underlying reason for lung volume loss. Collapse from a large pneumothorax is best treated with a chest tube. Suctioning or bronchoscopy should be used to treat atelectasis from mucus plugging or excessive secretions. Dependent atelectasis and lung consolidation are treated with PEEP augmentation, pulmonary recruitment, and positional change such as prone positioning. Typical recruitment maneuvers (RMs) consist of prolonged respiratory holds at increased airway pressures (eg, 30–40 second end-expiratory hold at 40 cm H_2O performed on a ventilator circuit) done in the absence of additional tidal breathing.

RMs are associated with improved Pao_2 but may adversely lower CO by decreasing venous return and increasing right-sided afterload. When performed, controlled RMs on a ventilator are the recommended approach. Both the beneficial and unwanted effects of RMs tend to be short-lived.[30] RMs can hyperinflate some lungs segments while simultaneously recruiting others and are less likely to benefit if hyperinflation predominates. In a small study of early ARDS patients, lung morphology seen on CT scan predicted a sustained improvement in oxygenation in patients with nonfocal ARDS versus focal disease.[31] A typical CT scan of focal ARDS shows posterior-dependent consolidation and atelectasis versus a more homogeneous pattern in nonfocal ARDS patients. Focal ARDS is more prone to hyperinflation without sustained improvement in oxygenation, suggesting that RMs are less likely to benefit patients with this ARDS morphology. Due to the heterogeneity among ARDS patients and lack of proved benefit, RMs should not be performed on a routine basis in all ARDS patients.[30] RMs may be helpful during life-threatening hypoxia but the potential risk and benefit should be assessed by the bedside provider on a case-by-case basis.

Neuromuscular blockade provides another means to improve oxygenation. Muscle relaxation improves gas exchange by eliminating ventilator dyssynchrony and facilitating alveolar recruitment. Early use of cisatracurium improves 28-day mortality in severe ARDS with P/F ratio less than 150.[32] The exact mechanism of benefit is unknown but may relate to improved respiratory mechanics leading to attenuation of systemic inflammatory mediators liberated during ventilation of severely injured lung.[33] The incidence of muscle weakness was not increased in the treatment group, suggesting that 2 days of neuromuscular blockade does not invoke significant adverse effects. Given these data, neuromuscular blockade is recommended in the emergency department for patients with P/F ratio less than 150, even in the absence of refractory hypoxemia.

Diffusion

Pulmonary oxygen diffusion capacity across the alveolar membrane is another target to improve pulmonary efficiency. In ARDS, diffusion improvements typically require alveolar fluid removal via active fluid management in the form of diuretics or ultrafiltration. A conservative fluid strategy compared with a liberal fluid strategy was associated with improved oxygenation, length of hospitalization, and ICU days without increase in other organ failures in a randomized trial of 1000 ARDS patients.[34] The general goals are to maintain a central venous pressure between 4 mm Hg and 8 mm Hg and a urine output greater than 0.5 mL/kg/h while simultaneously ensuring adequate CO.[34] Given these data, net fluid balance should be meticulously maintained in all patients with ARDS and shocked patients should be evaluated for volume responsiveness prior to empiric fluid loading whenever possible. Neutral to negative fluid balance should be the goal for all hemodynamically stable ARDS patients.

Redistribution of Blood Flow

Systemic blood flow (ie, CO) is another therapeutic target to rescue patients from life-threatening hypoxia. All ARDS patients should be screened for cardiac dysfunction because conditions causing ARDS can simultaneously induce myocardial dysfunction (affecting the left ventricle) and the high mean airway pressures associated with ARDS can reduce right ventricular performance.[12] If there is evidence of inadequate CO (elevated lactate, decreased mixed venous oxygen saturation [SvO_2], mottled skin, or low urine output) with abnormal cardiac performance, inotropic therapy may help optimize SvO_2 and consequently improve arterial oxygenation.

Blood flow can also be redistributed within the lung via inhaled pulmonary artery vasodilators and prone positioning. Inhaled nitric oxide (iNO) and inhaled epoprostenol selectively vasodilate the ventilated pulmonary artery beds, thereby improving ventilation to perfusion (V/Q) matching. iNO improves gas exchange in ARDS but unfortunately does not confer a mortality benefit.[35,36] The association of iNO and renal failure contributes to the conclusion that iNO should not be routinely used in ARDS. Patients with ARDS complicated by acute right ventricular failure have not specifically been studied. Use of iNO for rescue therapy in refractory hypoxemia or as a bridge to alternative therapies in patients at high risk of death from hypoxemia may be warranted on an individual basis.

Prone positioning, first described in 1976, is another method to improve gas exchange in ARDS. Prone positioning redistributes pulmonary blood flow to less consolidated anterior lung segments and improves gas exchange by improving V/Q matching. Mortality benefit was recently validated in ARDS patient with P/F ratio less than 150.[37] This trial enrolled patients after a 12- to 24-hour period of stabilization if the P/F ratio remained less than 150. The average Pao_2 in all the patients constantly increased during the first 4 hours of prone positioning and consistently decreased during periods of supine ventilation. Prone positioning reduces the need for other rescue therapies, such as ECMO, iNO, and high-frequency oscillatory ventilation (HFOV).[38] This procedure should be performed by personnel familiar with the specific complications. Procedures, such as central lines, nasogastric tubes, and chest tubes, should be performed prior to prone positioning. Prone ventilation is not consistently associated with an improvement in compliance, suggesting recruitment of healthy lung is not the only physiologic advantage.[37]

Extracorporeal Membrane Oxygenation

Venovenous-ECMO (VV-ECMO) maintains systemic gas exchange via a modified cardiopulmonary bypass circuit. Use of ECMO for severe refractory hypoxemia during the 2009 to 2010 influenza H1N1 pandemic highlights the viability of this specialized rescue therapy for patients with acute refractory disease.[39] ECMO is primarily used as a bridge to native lung recovery. In most cases, gas exchange via the ECMO circuit provides the opportunity for ultraprotective lung ventilation. The disadvantages of ECMO include hemorrhage due to the need for systemic anticoagulation and large vessel cannulation. Indications and contraindications for VV-ECMO are listed in **Table 6**.

Based on the results of the 2009 CESAR trial, patients with severe ARDS despite optimal medical therapy should be referred to an ECMO center. This trial randomized 180 adults with severe ARDS to either standard local care or referral to a specialized ECMO center. The primary outcome of disability free survival at 6 months was improved in the ECMO group and the therapy was deemed cost effective. This study has been criticized because not all of the patients in the intervention group received ECMO and only 70% of patients in the control group were treated with lung-protective ventilation.[40] It was pragmatically designed, however, to help determine the best real-life patient management strategy in severe ARDS. Referral to an ECMO center directly from an emergency department should be strongly considered for patients with early severe ARDS based on this trial.

MECHANICAL VENTILATION

Mechanical ventilation primarily aims to support gas exchange in critically ill patients. Mechanical ventilation in ARDS patients is more difficult due to risk of

Table 6
Extracorporeal membrane oxygenation indications and contraindications

Extracorporeal Membrane Oxygenation Usage for Acute Respiratory Distress Syndrome	
Indications	**Contraindications**
Consider ECMO if predicted mortality >50%	Condition prohibiting anticoagulation
Strongly consider for severe ARDS despite optimal medical management for 6 h	Recent central nervous system hemorrhage Nonrecoverable comorbidity Major pharmacologic immunosuppression Age >65 is relative contraindication

inducing or prolonging lung injury secondary to the ventilator induced damage. A useful analogy when dealing with ARDS patients is the baby lung principle,[6] which refers to the physiologic similarities between an ARDS lung and a miniature lung: ARDS-induced consolidation significantly reduces the effective lung volume capable of gas exchange. While manipulating the ventilator, it is helpful to adjust the perception of normal tidal volume for each particular patient. **Table 7** lists goals of mechanical ventilation among ARDS patients. The 2000 ARDSNet trial of low tidal volume ventilation is a landmark trial that redefined the standard of care for ARDS patients. It compared 6 mL/kg to 12 mL/kg of ideal body weight. There was a 9% absolute mortality benefit with the low-volume strategy despite lower oxygen levels during the first 24 hours. The advantage is likely related to reduced lung injury and systemic inflammation in the low tidal volume group. There have not been any head-to-head trials of 6 mL/kg compared with 8 mL/kg (common setting today for non-ARDS patients) but 6 mL/kg should be considered the proper starting point for all ARDS patients. The P/F threshold at which a low tidal volume strategy provides benefit is unclear and some experts propose an initial setting of 6 mL/kg for all ventilated patients, regardless of lung disease. This strategy for non-ARDS patients, however, may lead to more ventilator dysynchrony and increasing sedation requirements without much benefit.

One side effect of the low tidal volume strategy is reduced minute ventilation. Compensatory increase in respiratory rate is limited by expiratory time. Inadequate expiratory time must be avoided to prevent dynamic hyperinflation leading to auto-PEEP. Furthermore, the pathologic dead space associated with ARDS contributed to hypercapnia despite supranormal minute ventilation. Permissive hypercapnea during ARDS management is well tolerated and considered safe in most clinical scenarios, although patients with acute brain injury, arrhythmias, or right ventricular failure are possible exceptions. Hypercapnea also increases pulmonary vascular

Table 7	
Mechanical ventilation goals in acute respiratory distress syndrome	
Tidal volume	4–6 mL/kg of ideal body weight
Plateau pressure	Ideally <30 cm H_2O but lower may be better
pH, respiratory rate, minute ventilation	Depends on patient comorbidities but pH of 7.2 is widely accepted as acceptable permissive hypercapnia; lower may also be acceptable
PEEP	Unknown; higher may be better for severe ARDS
F_{IO_2}	Unknown; titration based on PEEP to F_{IO_2} table is appropriate

resistance. Although this is generally well tolerated, it may be a contributing factor in acute right ventricular failure during ARDS.

MODES OF VENTILATION

When changing modes of ventilation or ventilator settings in ARDS, the primary physiologic goal is supporting oxygenation via augmented mean airway pressure while maintaining a safe plateau pressure. In addition to the former consideration, lengthening inspiratory time helps achieve this goal. At extremes of prolonged inspiratory period, this is often referred to as inverse ratio ventilation. Inverse ratio ventilation may increase oxygenation but has not been shown to improve outcomes in ARDS patients. A majority of ARDS trials were conducted with volume control ventilation although pressure control ventilation is generally comparable, as long as the dependent variables are appropriately monitored in each mode.[41]

HFOV and airway pressure release ventilation represent the extreme of a prolonged inspiratory time strategy. HFOV has the theoretic advantage of safely maximizing the mean airway pressure because the mean airway pressure and plateau pressure are effectively the same. Unfortunately, early HFOV failed to show benefit in 2 randomized trials of ARDS patients and cannot be recommended as routine therapy in severe ARDS.[42,43] HFOV cannot be routinely recommended for severe ARDS patients but may have some value as rescue therapy in selected patients with severe ARDS failing other modalities.

MEDICATIONS

As discussed previously, early use of muscle relaxants provides a survival benefit for patients with ARDS and P/F ratio less than 150. Several other medications have been

Therapy	Pa_{O_2} to F_{IO_2} ratio		
	300–200	200–100	100–0
Prone positioning	Not recommended	Recommended	
6 cc/kg tidal volume	Recommended		
Cis-atricurium	Not Recommended	Recommended	
Plateau <30 cm H_2O	Recommended		
Increased PEEP	Not recommended	Recommended with caveats	
Conservative fluids	Recommended		
Recruitment Maneuvers	Only in case-by-case basis		
ECMO	Not recommended	Consider	
Inotropes	Maintaining adequate cardiac output is recommended at all ratios		
Esophageal guided PEEP	Encouraging but not enough data		
iNO	Not recommended		
HFOV	Not recommended and might be harmful		Possible rescue

Fig. 4. Guide to therapies for acute respiratory distress syndrome based on Pa_{O_2} to fraction of inspired oxygen ratio.

studied with no difference in outcomes. β-Agonists were studied in a multicenter, randomized, placebo-controlled trial and no clinically important differences were found.[44] Rosuvastatin was compared with placebo in 745 patients with ARDS from sepsis and did not show any improvement in mortality or ventilator-free days and there was actually an increase in kidney and liver dysfunction in the rosuvastatin group.[45]

SUMMARY

The summary of effective therapies for ARDS patients is listed in **Fig. 4**. All ARDS patients should be ventilated with a low-volume strategy aiming to maintain the plateau pressure less than 30 cm H_2O. Volume control ventilation is recommended, although pressure control ventilation and pressure-regulated volume control are also safe. Permissive hypercapnea to a pH of 7.20 is safe and may be protective. A conservative fluid strategy should be used for all ARDS patients not in shock. PEEP should probably be increased for patients with P/F ratio less than 200 although specific patient populations benefiting from this practice are not fully elucidated. For ARDS patients with P/F ratio less than 150, early neuromuscular blocking agents, prone positioning, and referral to an ECMO center have been shown to reduce mortality. β-Agonists, iNO, and HFOV have failed to show improvements in mortality or other clinically important endpoints and cannot be recommended.

ACKNOWLEDGMENTS

Special acknowledgment to Dr Holt Murray at the University of Pittsburgh Medical Center for his guidance on this article.

REFERENCES

1. Rubenfeld GD, Caldwell E, Peabody E, et al. Incidence and outcomes of acute lung injury. N Engl J Med 2005;353(16):1685–93.
2. Erickson SE, Martin GS, Davis JL, et al. Recent trends in acute lung injury mortality: 1996-2005. Crit Care Med 2009;37(5):1574–9.
3. Zambon M, Vincent JL. Mortality rates for patients with acute lung injury/ARDS have decreased over time. Chest 2008;133(5):1120–7.
4. Ranieri VM, Rubenfeld GD, Thompson BT, et al. Acute respiratory distress syndrome: the Berlin definition. JAMA 2012;307(23):2526–33.
5. Calandrino FS Jr, Anderson DJ, Mintun MA, et al. Pulmonary vascular permeability during the adult respiratory distress syndrome: a positron emission tomographic study. Am Rev Respir Dis 1988;138(2):421–8.
6. Gattinoni L, Pelosi P, Pesenti A, et al. CT scan in ARDS: clinical and physiopathological insights. Acta Anaesthesiol Scand Suppl 1991;95:87–94.
7. Aberle DR, Wiener-Kronish JP, Webb WR, et al. Hydrostatic versus increased permeability pulmonary edema: diagnosis based on radiographic criteria in critically ill patients. Radiology 1988;168(1):73–9.
8. Rana R, Vlahakis NE, Daniels CE, et al. B-type natriuretic peptide in the assessment of acute lung injury and cardiogenic pulmonary edema. Crit Care Med 2006;34(7):1941–6.
9. Rudiger A, Gasser S, Fischler M, et al. Comparable increase of B-type natriuretic peptide and amino-terminal pro-B-type natriuretic peptide levels in patients with severe sepsis, septic shock, and acute heart failure. Crit Care Med 2006;34(8):2140–4.

10. Roberts E, Ludman AJ, Dworzynski K, et al. The diagnostic accuracy of the natriuretic peptides in heart failure: systematic review and diagnostic meta-analysis in the acute care setting. BMJ 2015;350:h910.
11. Komiya K, Ishii H, Murakami J, et al. Comparison of chest computed tomography features in the acute phase of cardiogenic pulmonary edema and acute respiratory distress syndrome on arrival at the emergency department. J Thorac Imaging 2013;28(5):322–8.
12. Bouhemad B, Nicolas-Robin A, Arbelot C, et al. Acute left ventricular dilatation and shock-induced myocardial dysfunction. Crit Care Med 2009;37(2):441–7.
13. Copetti R, Soldati G, Copetti P. Chest sonography: a useful tool to differentiate acute cardiogenic pulmonary edema from acute respiratory distress syndrome. Cardiovasc Ultrasound 2008;6:16.
14. Ventilation with lower tidal volumes as compared with traditional tidal volumes for acute lung injury and the acute respiratory distress syndrome. The Acute Respiratory Distress Syndrome Network. N Engl J Med 2000; 342(18):1301–8.
15. Curley GF, Laffey JG, Kavanagh BP. CrossTalk proposal: there is added benefit to providing permissive hypercapnia in the treatment of ARDS. J Physiol 2013; 591(Pt 11):2763–5.
16. Kregenow DA, Rubenfeld GD, Hudson LD, et al. Hypercapnic acidosis and mortality in acute lung injury. Crit Care Med 2006;34(1):1–7.
17. Abdelsalam M. Permissive hypoxemia: is it time to change our approach? Chest 2006;129(1):210–1.
18. Rashkin MC, Bosken C, Baughman RP. Oxygen delivery in critically ill patients. Relationship to blood lactate and survival. Chest 1985;87(5):580–4.
19. Stapleton RD, Wang BM, Hudson LD, et al. Causes and timing of death in patients with ARDS. Chest 2005;128(2):525–32.
20. Wettstein RB, Shelledy DC, Peters JI. Delivered oxygen concentrations using low-flow and high-flow nasal cannulas. Respir Care 2005;50(5):604–9.
21. O'Reilly NA, Kelly PT, Stanton J, et al. Measurement of oxygen concentration delivered via nasal cannulae by tracheal sampling. Respirology 2014;19(4): 538–43.
22. Ritchie JE, Williams AB, Gerard C, et al. Evaluation of a humidified nasal high-flow oxygen system, using oxygraphy, capnography and measurement of upper airway pressures. Anaesth Intensive Care 2011;39(6):1103–10.
23. Li J, Murphy-Lavoie H, Bugas C, et al. Complications of emergency intubation with and without paralysis. Am J Emerg Med 1999;17(2):141–3.
24. Carroll GC. Misapplication of alveolar gas equation. N Engl J Med 1985; 312(9):586.
25. Brower RG, Lanken PN, MacIntyre N, et al. Higher versus lower positive end-expiratory pressures in patients with the acute respiratory distress syndrome. N Engl J Med 2004;351(4):327–36.
26. Meade MO, Cook DJ, Guyatt GH, et al. Ventilation strategy using low tidal volumes, recruitment maneuvers, and high positive end-expiratory pressure for acute lung injury and acute respiratory distress syndrome: a randomized controlled trial. JAMA 2008;299(6):637–45.
27. Briel M, Meade M, Mercat A, et al. Higher vs lower positive end-expiratory pressure in patients with acute lung injury and acute respiratory distress syndrome: systematic review and meta-analysis. JAMA 2010;303(9):865–73.
28. Amato MB, Meade MO, Slutsky AS, et al. Driving pressure and survival in the acute respiratory distress syndrome. N Engl J Med 2015;372(8):747–55.

29. Talmor D, Sarge T, Malhotra A, et al. Mechanical ventilation guided by esophageal pressure in acute lung injury. N Engl J Med 2008;359(20):2095–104.
30. Fan E, Wilcox ME, Brower RG, et al. Recruitment maneuvers for acute lung injury: a systematic review. Am J Respir Crit Care Med 2008;178(11):1156–63.
31. Constantin JM, Grasso S, Chanques G, et al. Lung morphology predicts response to recruitment maneuver in patients with acute respiratory distress syndrome. Crit Care Med 2010;38(4):1108–17.
32. Papazian L, Forel JM, Gacouin A, et al. Neuromuscular blockers in early acute respiratory distress syndrome. N Engl J Med 2010;363(12):1107–16.
33. Forel JM, Roch A, Marin V, et al. Neuromuscular blocking agents decrease inflammatory response in patients presenting with acute respiratory distress syndrome. Crit Care Med 2006;34(11):2749–57.
34. Wiedemann HP, Wheeler AP, Bernard GR, et al. Comparison of two fluid-management strategies in acute lung injury. N Engl J Med 2006;354(24):2564–75.
35. Adhikari NK, Burns KE, Friedrich JO, et al. Effect of nitric oxide on oxygenation and mortality in acute lung injury: systematic review and meta-analysis. BMJ 2007;334(7597):779.
36. Adhikari NK, Dellinger RP, Lundin S, et al. Inhaled nitric oxide does not reduce mortality in patients with acute respiratory distress syndrome regardless of severity: systematic review and meta-analysis. Crit Care Med 2014;42(2):404–12.
37. Guerin C, Reignier J, Richard JC, et al. Prone positioning in severe acute respiratory distress syndrome. N Engl J Med 2013;368(23):2159–68.
38. Gattinoni L, Taccone P, Carlesso E, et al. Prone position in acute respiratory distress syndrome. Rationale, indications, and limits. Am J Respir Crit Care Med 2013;188(11):1286–93.
39. Noah MA, Peek GJ, Finney SJ, et al. Referral to an extracorporeal membrane oxygenation center and mortality among patients with severe 2009 influenza A(H1N1). JAMA 2011;306(15):1659–68.
40. Peek GJ, Mugford M, Tiruvoipati R, et al. Efficacy and economic assessment of conventional ventilatory support versus extracorporeal membrane oxygenation for severe adult respiratory failure (CESAR): a multicentre randomised controlled trial. Lancet 2009;374(9698):1351–63.
41. Esteban A, Alia I, Gordo F, et al. Prospective randomized trial comparing pressure-controlled ventilation and volume-controlled ventilation in ARDS. For the Spanish Lung Failure Collaborative Group. Chest 2000;117(6):1690–6.
42. Young D, Lamb SE, Shah S, et al. High-frequency oscillation for acute respiratory distress syndrome. N Engl J Med 2013;368(9):806–13.
43. Ferguson ND, Cook DJ, Guyatt GH, et al. High-frequency oscillation in early acute respiratory distress syndrome. N Engl J Med 2013;368(9):795–805.
44. Matthay MA, Brower RG, Carson S, et al. Randomized, placebo-controlled clinical trial of an aerosolized beta(2)-agonist for treatment of acute lung injury. Am J Respir Crit Care Med 2011;184(5):561–8.
45. Truwit JD, Bernard GR, Steingrub J, et al. Rosuvastatin for sepsis-associated acute respiratory distress syndrome. N Engl J Med 2014;370(23):2191–200.

Management of Acute Exacerbation of Asthma and Chronic Obstructive Pulmonary Disease in the Emergency Department

Salvador J. Suau, MD*, Peter M.C. DeBlieux, MD

KEYWORDS

• Asthma • Asthmatic crisis • COPD • AECOPD

KEY POINTS

• Management of severe asthma and chronic obstructive pulmonary disease (COPD) exacerbations require similar medical interventions in the acute care setting.
• Capnography, electrocardiography, chest x-ray, and ultrasonography are important diagnostic tools in patients with undifferentiated shortness of breath.
• Bronchodilators and corticosteroids are first-line therapies for both asthma and COPD exacerbations.
• Noninvasive ventilation, magnesium, and ketamine should be considered in patients with severe symptoms and in those not responding to first-line therapy.
• A detailed plan reviewed with the patient before discharge can decrease the number of future exacerbations.

INTRODUCTION

Acute asthma and chronic obstructive pulmonary disease (COPD) exacerbations are the most common respiratory diseases requiring emergent medical evaluation and treatment. Asthma accounts for more than 2 million visits to emergency departments (EDs), and approximately 4000 annual deaths in the United States.[1] In a similar fashion, COPD is a major cause of morbidity and mortality. It affects more than 14.2 million Americans (±9.8 million who may be undiagnosed).[2] COPD accounts for more than 1.5 million yearly ED visits and is the fourth leading cause of death

Disclosures: None.
Louisiana State University, University Medical Center of New Orleans, 2000 Canal Street, D&T 2nd Floor - Suite 2720, New Orleans, LA 70112, USA
* Corresponding author.
E-mail address: ssuau@lsuhsc.edu

Emerg Med Clin N Am 34 (2016) 15–37
http://dx.doi.org/10.1016/j.emc.2015.08.002
0733-8627/16/$ – see front matter © 2016 Elsevier Inc. All rights reserved.
emed.theclinics.com

worldwide.[3,4] Both asthma and COPD exacerbations impose an enormous economic burden on the US health care budget with estimates of more than $56 billion annually for asthma,[5] and $49.9 billion annually for COPD.[4] A recent study found that, despite significant efforts to educate the public and increase disease awareness, the rates of COPD hospitalizations have increased by 20% to 30% between 2002 and 2012. The inpatient monetary charges for these hospitalizations have increased by an alarming 125%, and the rate of hospital readmissions for patients with poorly controlled COPD remains at 21%.[6]

Asthma and COPD are chronic, debilitating disease processes that have been differentiated traditionally by the presence or absence of reversible airflow obstruction. In daily clinical practice, it is difficult to differentiate these 2 obstructive processes based on their symptoms, and on their nearly identical acute treatment strategies. Their major differences are important only when discussing anatomic sites involved, long-term prognosis, and the nature of inflammatory markers. These aspects affect disease response to certain pharmacologic treatment options.[7]

DEFINITIONS

The Global Initiative for Asthma (GINA) described asthma as an allergic disease, typically commencing in childhood,[2,8] and characterized by increased bronchial hyperresponsiveness, increased vascular permeability, bronchial smooth muscle spasm, and the release of inflammatory mediators. This pathophysiology translates into recurrent episodes of wheezing, difficulty breathing, chest tightness, and coughing.[9]

Asthma exacerbations are variable and episodic. Asthma can be triggered by a plethora of environmental agents, infectious precipitants, emotional or exercise states, and diverse exposure to ingested or inhaled agents, typically resolving completely either spontaneously or with treatment.[8,10]

The Global Initiative for Chronic Obstructive Lung Disease (GOLD) guidelines define COPD as an acquired and preventable disease resulting primarily from tobacco smoking, and characterized by persistent airflow obstruction, and decline in progressive lung function.[2,4] It usually develops after the fourth decade of life, and it is characterized by shortness of breath, cough, and sputum production.[4] The airflow limitations are classically progressive and associated with an abnormal inflammatory response to diverse inhaled agents, gases, and particles.[7]

PATHOPHYSIOLOGY

There is not strong evidence suggesting histopathologic overlap between these 2 obstructive entities, known as the asthma–COPD overlap syndrome.[2] The most important pathologic difference between asthma and COPD is the inflammatory cells that mediate each respective disease process. Eosinophils and CD4 cells mainly mediate asthma, whereas neutrophils and CD8 cells mediate COPD.[2] This basic difference allows inhaled corticosteroids (CS) to be more efficacious against eosinophilic-mediated asthma, and largely ineffective against the primarily neutrophilic inflammation seen in COPD.[2,7] Regardless of their pathologic differences or their similar inciting agents, it is paramount that emergent risk stratification and treatment modalities be initiated expeditiously to decrease clinical deterioration, morbidity, and mortality.

RISK STRATIFICATION

Risk stratification of the severely short of breath (SOB) patient requires several steps and can be a difficult feat when an undifferentiated patient with SOB presents to the

ED. The practitioner should undertake a methodologic approach to optimize the acquisition of a pertinent history and quickly determine the best management pathway. **Box 1** provides some high-yield questions that will aid in the initial assessment of the dyspneic patient.[4,11]

After these initial questions, the severity of the exacerbation can be assessed with objective physical findings such as vital signs, including oxygen saturation, heart rate (HR), and respiratory rate; degree of wheezing and air movement; use of accessory muscles; degree of difficulty with speech; peak expiratory flow; and end-tidal carbon dioxide ($ETCO_2$) monitoring.[4,11] It is imperative to understand that the absence of severity markers does not exclude the presence of a life-threatening disease process. A helpful algorithm to aid in differentiating between mild, moderate, and severe exacerbation is presented in **Fig. 1**.

The final step during the primary assessment of the patient with SOB is the essential consideration that wheezing and respiratory distress can also be found in multiple other disease states. An adequate differential diagnosis must be formulated to prevent the creation of an anchoring bias, which would prevent a clinician from maintaining a broad differential diagnosis. **Box 2** illustrates a differential diagnosis of wheezing in adults and children.

ACUTE DECOMPENSATED HEART FAILURE

The acutely undifferentiated patient with SOB may have multiple comorbidities that might contribute or disguise the exact inciting disease process. Two commonly encountered examples are heart failure (HF) and COPD. These 2 entities are frequently encountered in the elderly and tobacco smoker. Several studies estimate the prevalence of HF in COPD patients to be somewhere between 20% and 30%.[12] Similar studies have also reported that the presence of HF in COPD is associated with worse clinical outcomes.[13,14]

DIAGNOSIS
Spirometry

GOLD, GINA, and other evidenced-based guidelines have been developed as blueprints for the identification, prevention, and treatment of both these obstructive

---

Box 1
Important risk factors in the asthmatic/COPD patient

- Previous endotracheal intubations
- Previous intensive care unit admissions
- ≥2 non-ICU hospitalizations in the past 1 year
- ≥3 ED visits in the past month
- Chronic use of oral corticosteroids
- Medication noncompliance
- Living in poverty with no access to health care
- Using ≥2 SABA pressurized metered dose inhalers monthly

Abbreviations: COPD, chronic obstructive pulmonary disease; ED, emergency department; ICU, intensive care unit; SABA, short-acting β-agonist.

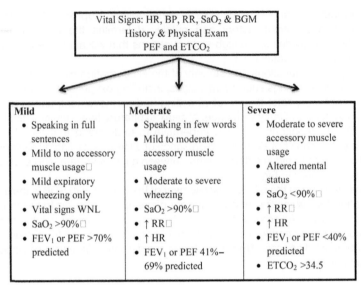

Fig. 1. Dyspneic exacerbation severity algorithm. BGM, blood glucose monitor; BP, blood pressure; $ETCO_2$, end-tidal carbon dioxide; FEV_1, forced expiratory volume in 1 second; HR, heart rate; PEF, peak expiratory flow; RR, respiratory rate; WNL, within normal limits.

entities. Both GOLD and GINA recommend baseline spirometry to diagnose and classify these diseases.[4,8] Despite this standard recommendation, there is no clinical benefit to performing spirometry in the acute care setting. Spirometry is not a suitable tool for the emergent management of the undifferentiated dyspneic patient.

Box 2	
Differential diagnosis of wheezing	
Adults	**Children**
• Upper respiratory tract infection	• Upper respiratory tract infection
• Pneumonia	• Croup
• Asthma	• Tracheomalasia
• Chronic obstructive pulmonary disease	• Bronchiolitis
• Congestive heart failure	• Asthma
• Chronic bronchitis	• Pneumonia
• Gastroesophageal reflux disease	• Foreign body
• Acute coronary syndrome	
• Pulmonary embolism	
• Foreign body	
• Pneumothorax	
• Cystic fibrosis	
• Vocal cord dysfunction	

Laboratory Tests

There is currently no laboratory test that will specifically identify asthma or acute exacerbations of COPD (AECOPD) as the etiology of the acutely patient with SOB. Any standard serum laboratory studies should only be drawn to assist in deciphering the etiology of the acute decompensation. Sputum testing is unreliable and should not be gathered, unless tuberculosis is suspected as the underlying etiology of the exacerbation. GOLD only recommends sputum testing in the AECOPD patient who has failed initial antibiotic therapy.[4] Viruses are strongly associated with AECOPD; therefore, testing for influenza may provide important implications in management of these patients.[15]

Blood Gas Analysis

Arterial blood gas analysis is a routine test performed in the severe asthmatic and AECOPD patient. Several guidelines recommend its use in moderate and severe respiratory exacerbations: when the pulse oxygen saturation (SaO_2) is less than 92% on room air; and to follow pH, partial pressure of carbon dioxide (Pco_2), and partial pressure of oxygen. One must question the benefit of an arterial over a venous blood gas given the pain severity, the possibility of aneurysmal formation, arterial laceration, infection, and infrequently, the loss of limb.[16–26] These possible risks of the procedure must be coupled with the understanding that a normal Pco_2 in a venous blood gas analysis excludes arterial hypercarbia, making this painful and possibly complicated procedure unnecessary.[16–26]

Capnography

$ETCO_2$ during an AECOPD may be useful in the risk stratification of these patients. Doğan and colleagues[27] found that, when measuring with mainstream capnography devices, $ETCO_2$ levels were higher in admitted patients than those who were discharged from the ED. These levels must be obtained before any bronchodilator treatment. After the first bronchodilator treatment was completed, the $ETCO_2$ between the 2 groups showed no difference. This study also showed a strong correlation between $ETCO_2$ and arterial Pco_2, previously demonstrated by Cinar and colleagues.[28]

Electrocardiogram

Electrocardiography is an essential component in the acute evaluation of the patient with SOB. Part of the reported 58% increased mortality of patients with COPD between 1990 and 2010 has been linked to adverse cardiovascular events.[29] Although the exact pathophysiologic link remains unclear, data suggest that this could be caused partly by cardiac dysrhythmias.[30,31] **Fig. 2** demonstrates commonly encountered ECG changes that may be found in the AECOPD. These changes can be attributed to the clockwise rotation of the heart and the right atrial and ventricular hypertrophy that is seen in the COPD patient. Furthermore, P-wave verticalization is likely caused by the downward displacement of the heart owing to the progressive flattening of the diaphragms. This pathology is owing to the right atrium being physically anchored to the diaphragm by a strong aponeurosis.[32]

Other ECG findings in COPD include:

- S waves in leads I, II, and III;
- R/S ratio less than 1 in leads V5 or V6; and
- The lead I sign—isoelectric P wave, QRS amplitude less than 1.5 mm, and T wave amplitude less than 0.5 mm in lead I.

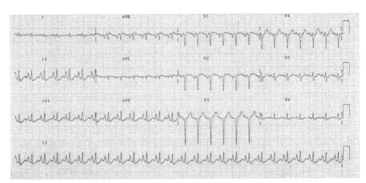

Fig. 2. (1) Tachycardia. Multifocal atrial tachycardia is rare, but specific to chronic obstructive pulmonary disease (COPD).[33] (2) Right axis deviation. (3) P wave axis of greater than 60° (considered to be 96% sensitive for COPD.[34]) (4) Low-voltage QRS amplitude in I, aVL, V5-V6. (May be found in leads II, III, or aVF [<5 mm]). (5) P pulmonale (peaked P waves in leads II, III, or aVF [>2.5 mm]). (*From* Burns E. The ECG in chronic obstructive pulmonary disease. Life in the Fast Lane. 2012. Available at: http://lifeinthefastlane.com/ecg-library/copd/. Accessed May 29, 2015. Life in the Fast Lane is licensed under a Creative Commons ShareAlike 4.0 International User's License http://creativecommons.org/licenses/by-sa/4.0/.)

If these criteria seem overly complex, a more simplified diagnostic marker is finding a P wave in lead aVL, or the P wave amplitude in lead III greater than in lead I.[35]

Radiography

The posteroanterior and lateral chest radiograph is the most widely used imaging modality in the evaluation of the acutely dyspneic patient. Typical findings include a flattened diaphragm, an increased anteroposterior diameter, an enlarged retrosternal airspace, a narrow vertical cardiac silhouette, and bullae.[36] Although none of these findings is diagnostic, a chest x-ray is more importantly obtained to rule out other causes of shortness of breath, such as pneumothorax, pulmonary infiltrates, or pulmonary edema. Tsai and colleagues[37] found that 21% of patients had their management altered by an initial chest x-ray. Pulmonary embolism has been found in 3% of COPD patients presenting to the ED.[38]

Chest radiography should be considered routine in the patient with an AECOPD. In patients with established asthma, there is more room for clinical judgment, and practitioners should consider a chest x-ray in patients who (1) are in extremis, (2) have clinical markers of pneumonia or pneumothorax, (3) are not responding to conventional therapy, (4) are presenting with new onset wheezing, and presumed de novo asthma, and (5) are at risk for an alternative diagnosis, for example, HF in the older adult and foreign body aspiration in the young child with wheezing.

Ultrasonography

Cardiopulmonary ultrasonography has become an important diagnostic tool in the ED setting because it decreases exposure to radiation. Three main protocols have come into favor. These include Lung Ultrasound in the Critically Ill (LUCI), Bedside Lung Ultrasonography in Emergency (BLUE), and Fluid Administration Limited by Lung Sonography (FULL).[39] Gallard and colleagues[40] found that ultrasonography has an accuracy of 95% in diagnosing COPD or asthma exacerbations. This reinforced the findings of Silva and colleagues,[41] who found a 92% accuracy of ultrasonography in diagnosing these conditions.

TREATMENT
Oxygen

Oxygen therapy is a key feature in the management of an undifferentiated patient with SOB. In an acute asthma exacerbation, GINA and the British Thoracic Society recommend that oxygen be the first-line treatment. They strongly emphasize this recommendation with the understanding that hypoxia must be addressed expeditiously and oxygen administration should be monitored closely for efficacy. This differs significantly from their guidelines for the AECOPD patient. The Fio_2 provided to this patient population should be no greater than 28%. Bronchodilators are to be given with compressed air rather than oxygen. These recommendations stem from the knowledge that hyperoxia leads to decreased minute ventilation and hypercapnia.[42] Such increases in carbon dioxide are more likely to be seen in older patients and those with a home oxygen dependence, and can cause neurologic and cardiac depression.[43]

Austin and colleagues[44] showed a reduced mortality in COPD patients with titrated oxygen therapy. Oxygen administration guidelines should therefore be in place in both the prehospital setting as well as in the ED. Oxygen can be titrated according to a saturation of peripheral oxygen (SpO_2), with no oxygen given at an SpO_2 of greater than 92%, 2 to 3 L via nasal cannula at an SpO_2 of 85% to 92%, and a face mask with higher flows used for an SpO_2 of less than 85%.[45] An arterial blood gas can then be obtained to further guide oxygen requirements.

Bronchodilators

The first-line pharmacotherapy in the emergent management of the asthmatic crisis and AECOPD is the administration of bronchodilators.[46] These agents target the bronchial hyperactivity and attempt to reverse, or ameliorate airflow obstruction. Although COPD is usually considered an irreversible process, most acute COPD exacerbations have a reversible component that must be targeted. The primary pharmacotherapy agents used are short-acting β2-agonists (SABA) and ipratropium bromide.

Short-acting β2-receptor agonists

SABA relax pulmonary smooth muscle by stimulating airway $β_2$-adrenergic receptors, increasing intracellular cyclic adenosine monophosphate. This increase in cyclic adenosine monophosphate inhibits smooth muscle bronchoconstriction. SABA's typical time of onset is seconds to minutes, with peak effect at 30 minutes and a half-life of 4 to 6 hours.[4,8] The most widely used SABA is albuterol, a racemic mixture of 2 enantiomers, namely (R)-albuterol and (S)-albuterol. (R)-albuterol is the active form, binding to β2-receptors and provides the desired bronchodilation. This also causes the more undesired, tachycardia, tremors, and anxiety/restlessness. (S)-albuterol, the inert form, is hypothesized to possibly have detrimental effects on airway function.[46] This was the premise of the development of levalbuterol, a purified version of the (R)-albuterol enantiomer that was marketed as having fewer of the unwanted cardiac adverse effects than racemic albuterol. Multiple studies have shown that continuous nebulized levalbuterol is not superior to continuous nebulized albuterol and that levalbuterol had no beneficial effects on HR.[47,48] In a metaanalysis of 7 clinical trials conducted by Jat and Khairwa,[49] there was no evidence supporting the theory that levalbuterol is superior to albuterol regarding efficacy and patient safety.

Long-acting β2-receptor agonists

Long-acting $β_2$-receptor agonists (LABAs) such as salmeterol and formoterol were widely used in the early 1990s because they provided approximately 12 hours of bronchodilation. In 1993, Castle and colleagues[50] showed significant evidence that salmeterol had a 3-fold mortality increase in asthmatic patients. This finding was quickly confirmed in 1996 by the US Food and Dug Administration's Salmeterol Multi-centre Asthma Research Trial (SMART). The study had to be prematurely stopped owing to increased exacerbations and mortality.[51] An additional study performed by Mann and colleagues[52] also demonstrated increased asthma exacerbations.

This is in contrast with current recommendations provided by the American College of Chest Physicians and the Canadian Thoracic Society to prevent AECOPD. LABAs have been shown to improve quality of life and lung function while decreasing moderate and severe exacerbations in COPD patients. Rate of adverse events and mortality were not increased compared with placebo in this patient population.[53] A LABA combined with an inhaled CS is preferable to monotherapy with either agent.

Anticholinergics

Inhaled ipratropium bromide (Atrovent) elicits its bronchodilatory effect by competitively inhibiting the muscarinic acetylcholine receptors of the pulmonary smooth muscle. Its time of onset is approximately 15 minutes, with a peak effect at 60 to 90 minutes and half-life of 6 to 8 hours, making it slower in onset and longer in duration than SABA.[54] This explains the common practice of using these inhaled agents in combination. The GOLD guidelines recommend a SABA as a first-line agent owing to its faster onset of action, followed by anticholinergics if a prompt response is not attained clinically.[4] The authors of this article agree with the findings of Vézina and colleagues,[55] who found that combined pharmacotherapy is more effective in decreasing ED admissions with no evidence of adverse effects. Ipratropium bromide can also be considered as a good alternative in patients who are intolerant of SABA side effects. The agent has been linked to lower ED admission rates in acutely severe exacerbations and may decrease the overall ED duration of stay.[56–58] A similar, but longer-acting antimuscarinic, tiotropium, has been shown to be an effective maintenance bronchodilator in both COPD and asthma patients. Kerstjens and associates[59] demonstrated that tiotropium improved symptomatic control in patients with poorly controlled symptoms who were on inhaled CS and LABAs and reduced severe exacerbations by 21%. In the first 24 hours of the respiratory obstructive crisis, some believe that the adrenergic receptors, which constitute the majority of pulmonary airway receptors, are downregulated and perhaps temporarily unresponsive to β_2-receptor agonists. During this time, pulmonary muscarinic acetylcholine receptors remain functional leading to their contribution in bronchodilation.[60–62]

Delivery mode

Method of pharmacotherapy delivery is via a pressurized metered dose inhaler with a holding chamber or an oxygen-driven nebulizer. The current literature does not show any difference in outcomes based on route of administration, except for slightly shorter ED duration of stay in those treated with gas-driven nebulizers.[63,64]

Magnesium sulfate

Intravenous (IV) magnesium sulfate ($MgSO_4$) is suggested to produce pulmonary smooth muscle relaxation via calcium receptor blockade or by activation of adenyl cyclase at the smooth muscle cellular level.[65] Regardless of its mechanism of action, its efficacy on the acute asthmatic crisis or the AECOPD remains uncertain, despite guidelines like GINA and GOLD advocating its use.[4,8] Two studies were recently undertaken to ascertain this agent's efficacy. The first, conducted by Goodacre and colleagues,[66] failed to show that either IV or nebulized $MgSO_4$ provided any clinically relevant benefit in adults with severe acute asthma. On the contrary, a second study performed by Kew and colleagues[67] found that IV $MgSO_4$ reduced hospital admissions and improved lung function when other pharmacotherapy had failed to ameliorate the acute exacerbation.

Corticosteroids

CS treatment is also considered first-line in the emergent management of the asthmatic crisis and AECOPD. CS have a complex mechanism of action that ultimately leads to the inhibition of potent inflammatory mediators and the reduction of airway inflammation. A recent Cochrane review conducted by Walters and colleagues[68] demonstrated that the use of CS was associated with a greater than 50% reduction in treatment failure. The number of patients needed to treat with CS to prevent 1 treatment failure was 9. This same study also showed that CS provided a 30-day relapse rate reduction, and a shorter hospital duration of stay, despite no association with decreased mortality.[68] The choice of which systemic CS (SCS) to use has been debated, and common practice dictates the use of glucocorticoids (prednisone, prednisolone, or methylprednisolone), because they are the most widely studied making them the preferred choice over SCS with mineralocorticoid effects like hydrocortisone.[69] There is still ongoing research regarding the most appropriate dose, route of administration, and duration of therapy. Currently, there is good consensus that there is no inferiority between oral and parenteral treatment with regards to rates of treatment failure, relapse rate, and mortality.[68,70] Therefore, if the patient can tolerate an oral agent, provide therapy orally and reserve parenteral treatment for those patients who cannot tolerate oral treatment.

Of note, a new pilot study conducted by Mendes and colleagues[71] regarding the emerging use of inhaled CS showed that, in adults with airflow obstruction, a single standard dose of an inhaled CS provided simultaneously with inhaled albuterol acutely potentiated the effects of the albuterol-induced pulmonary smooth muscle relaxation and increased the forced expiratory volume in 1 second (FEV_1) response versus the standard method.

Initial CS dosages have also been a topic of great debate secondary to the misconception that severity of disease warrants higher dosages of treatment. In 2013, Cheng and colleagues[72] performed a metaanalysis of 12 studies totaling 1172 patients; they were not able to demonstrate any benefit to CS dosages of greater than 80 mg/d. These findings were consistent with Alia and colleagues's[73] study from 2011, which demonstrated that SCS dosages of 0.5 mg/kg every 6 hours were sufficient, and higher dosages were unwarranted for achieving clinical outcomes. For example, higher dosages did not have decreased duration of stay, decreased length of ventilation, or decreased treatment failure with noninvasive ventilation (NIV). Despite no benefit found in larger dosages of SCS therapy, Schacke and colleagues[74,75] have shown that the risk of adverse effects increases with increased doses of CS. The main adverse reactions with larger doses of CS were hyperglycemia, myopathies, neurologic effects like anxiety and delirium, increased rate of infection, hypertension, and gastrointestinal bleeding.[74,75] These adverse effects were also documented by Kiser and colleagues,[76] who found the association of increased rates of hyperglycemia, need for insulin therapy, and increased rates of invasive fungal infections in patients that were given CS doses of greater than 240 mg/d. Dosages of greater than 2 mg/kg per day do not provide any clinical benefit, and will likely provide greater side effects in the management of the critically ill asthmatics or AECOPD.

The last vastly debated concept in CS treatment is the duration of treatment therapy. The literature has described a wide range of therapy from 5 days to 8 weeks. The Reduction in the Use of Corticosteroids in Exacerbated COPD (REDUCE) trial conducted by Leuppi and colleagues[77] demonstrated that short-term therapy was noninferior to a longer duration. It showed no difference in mortality, rate of relapse, or change in recovery of lung function based on treatment duration.[77]

Upon completion of these initial interventions, any additional treatment is based on the patient's clinical status. **Fig. 3** provides a suggested treatment algorithm for patients with severe asthma.[78] It can also serve as a helpful algorithm in the treatment of AECOPD.

Antibiotics

Antimicrobial pharmacotherapy is perhaps the only emergent treatment recommendation that will differ between the asthmatic and the AECOPD. As opposed to an asthmatic event, it is estimated that approximately 8 of every 10 AECOPD episodes precipitated by a pulmonary infection, with either a bacterial, viral, or fungal pathogen.[79–81] Furthermore, these authors estimate that 50% of the microbial-induced exacerbations are attributed to a bacterial pathogen, warranting antibiotic therapy. White and colleagues[82] have also suggested that antibiotic therapy in an AECOPD will decrease the risk of progression to pneumonia and will catalyze bacterial eradication that in turn will improve airway inflammation in the acute exacerbation. Macrolides are the best class of antibiotics class for the treatment of AECOPD. Martinez and colleagues[83] determined that macrolides have added antiinflammatory and immunomodulatory effects, in addition to their antibacterial efficacy. Barnes[84] has postulated that macrolide therapy may increase the pulmonary smooth muscle's response to CS via the increased recruitment of the enzyme histone deacetylase 2 that is integral in the inflammatory response seen in COPD patients. Finally, although macrolides may have additional benefits over other classes of antibiotics, if an allergic reaction develops, other commonly used agents such as β-lactams and fluoroquinolones are deemed appropriate alternatives.[84]

Noninvasive Ventilation

The airway management of a decompensating asthmatic and COPD patient must be monitored meticulously and prompt changes must be made if first-line therapy is not ameliorating the respiratory crisis. The early recognition and appropriate modification in management may prevent further decompensation and increased mortality. Carson and colleagues[85] report that patients who are decompensating warrant NIV. NIV is the mainstay of therapy in the acute management of most reversible respiratory emergencies. This treatment modality is best provided via full facial mask, although other delivery methods are available. It is postulated that NIV is a direct bronchodilator.[86] NIV also recruits alveoli secondary to external positive end expiratory pressure (PEEP), offsetting intrinsic PEEP.[87] Alveolar recruitment improves ventilation–perfusion mismatch by preventing airway closure and reducing the work of breathing.[88] NIV can be used for short periods of time as deemed clinically necessary and carries a lower risk of nosocomial pneumonia than endotracheal intubation (ETI).[89] **Fig. 3** suggests starting inspiratory positive airway pressure and expiratory positive airway pressure at 8 cm H_2O and 3 cm H_2O, respectively. The authors of this article strongly encourage that the practitioner remain at the patient's bedside directly monitoring work of breathing and serially increasing both inspiratory positive airway pressure and expiratory positive airway pressure to higher pressures within a 30 minute trial to optimize nebulizer and overall treatment time. A recent Cochrane review indicated that patients with acute asthma exacerbation who were treated with NIV had decreased admission rates, decreased duration of ICU stay, and an overall shorter hospital stay, although there was no clear benefit for reduced ETI or mortality.[90] Last, NIV has been shown to be safe in pregnant patients and in pediatric populations.[85] Relative contraindications include facial or

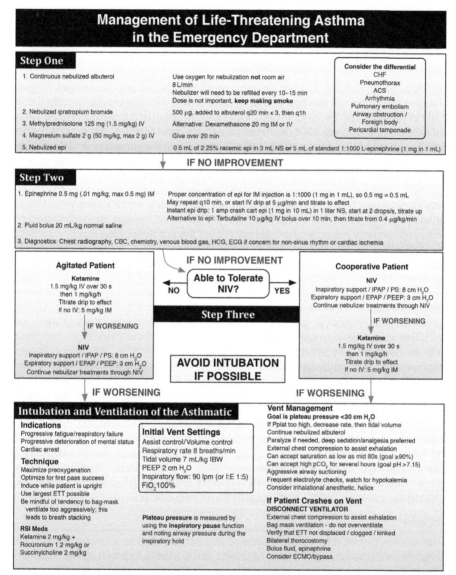

Fig. 3. Suggested treatment algorithm for patients with severe asthma. ACS, acute coronary syndrome; CBC, complete blood count; CHF, congestive heart failure; ECG, electrocardiograph; ECMO, extracorporeal membrane oxygenation; EPAP, expiratory positive airway pressure; ETT, endotracheal tube; epi, epinephrine; FiO_2, fraction of inspired oxygen; IBW, ideal body weight; IM, intramuscular; IPAP, inspiratory positive airway pressure; IV, intravenous; NIV, noninvasive monitoring; NS, normal saline; pCO_2, partial pressure of carbon dioxide; PEEP, positive end expiratory pressure; Pplat, airway plateau pressure; PS, pressure support. (*Courtesy of RJ Strayer, P Andrus, R. Arntfield and emupdates.com; used with permission.*)

esophageal trauma or surgery, deformities of the upper airway, copious secretions, or an uncooperative patient. Absolute contraindications are cardiac or respiratory arrest.[91]

High-Flow Nasal Cannula Oxygen Therapy

High-flow nasal cannula oxygen therapy provides heated and humidified oxygen through a nasal cannula at a flow rate of up to 60 L/min. It can be used as an alternative to NIV in patients who have poor tolerance to facial masks, and is helpful in asthmatics and COPD patients because it decreases anatomic dead space.[92] Although it cannot actively enhance tidal volume, the high flow increases airway pressure and decreases some the resistance of expiratory flow. The end-expiratory lung volume is also increased with an effect more pronounced in patients with a high body mass index.[93] High-flow nasal cannula oxygen therapy has also been found to provide better thoracoabdominal synchrony than with a facemask NIV. Unlike with a conventional nasal cannula, at high flows the actual inspiratory fraction of oxygen (Fio_2) delivered by the high-flow nasal cannula better approximates the predicted Fio_2.

Heliox

Heliox is a compound mixture of 80% helium and 20% oxygen. It can also be considered as an adjuvant in the early management of asthma before oxygen saturation requirements become the deciding parameter. Helium is a chemically inert, odorless, tasteless, noncombustible gas that has a lower molecular density than oxygen and air.[94] This lower density can serve as a better transport modality than traditional room air or 100% oxygen-driven nebulizers for the penetration of bronchodilating, anticholinergic, and antiinflammatory agents. It has been shown that heliox-driven bronchodilation brings about more rapid and greater improvement in FEV_1, forced vital capacity, and maximal expiratory flow rate than the traditional nebulizer methods.[95] Therefore, in asthmatic and AECOPD patients with an FEV_1 of 50% or less, helioxdriven nebulization treatments lead to better spirometry measurements than do airdriven nebulization treatments.[94] The most recent metaanalysis performed by Rodrigo and Rodriguez-Castro[96] in 2014 showed that β_2-agonist heliox-driven nebulization lowered the rate of ED admissions from 36% to 25% versus standard oxygendriven nebulization. This metaanalysis warrants additional prospective testing and comparison between heliox- and oxygen-driven nebulization.

Ketamine

Ketamine is a potent dissociative analgesic that can be used as a rescue agent in patients who have severe asthma and AECOPD that are refractory to first-line treatment options. It is characterized by an onset of action within 60 seconds, peak tissue distribution within 7 to 11 minutes, and an hepatic excretion half-life of 2 to 3 hours.[97] Ketamine holds several properties that can aid the AECOPD and severely asthmatic patient. First, ketamine has been shown to block the activation of N-methyl-D-aspartic acid (NMDA) receptors in the lung parenchyma. These NMDA receptors are responsible for stimulating the unwanted pulmonary edema and bronchoconstriction found during an AECOPD and in an asthmatic crisis.[98] Second, in the lung, ketamine has been found to downregulate production of the nitric oxide that is responsible for bronchospasm.[99] Third, ketamine has been found to block the recruitment of macrophages, interfere with cytokine production, and decrease interleukin-4 concentrations. These mechanisms are responsible for unwanted inflammatory changes, airway hyperreactivity, and bronchoconstriction in the acutely severe asthmatic patient.[100] All of these properties, along with the previously discussed upregulation of catecholamine levels and the anticholinergic effects on bronchial smooth muscle, argue strongly for ketamine as an advantageous adjuvant agent in the management of the AECOPD and decompensating asthmatic. Last, it is important to emphasize that ketamine, like all analgesic, amnestic, anesthetic, and muscle relaxants, be administered in a monitored environment where SaO_2, $ETCO_2$, blood pressure (BP), HR, and appropriate nursing presence is available continuously.

Epinephrine

Perhaps the most underappreciated and underused pharmacotherapy in our armamentarium for the treatment of an asthmatic crisis and the AECOPD is epinephrine. Some iconic practitioners would strongly argue that this agent should be placed on the top of every first-line treatment algorithm published by medical societies, a sentiment that both authors of this article share. The concern for a possible adverse cardiovascular event, increased risk of hypertension in an already uncontrolled hypertensive patient and the possible risk of aggravating the tachycardic state in an already tachycardic patient has placed this previously first-line agent at the bottom, if not completely off treatment algorithms. In 1988, Cydulka and colleagues[101] stated that, despite concerns of old age, concerns of potential adverse cardiac events, or concerns of increased risk of exacerbating BP and HR, epinephrine, dosed at starting doses of 0.3 mg of 1:1000 solution, did not cause any of these adverse reactions. Epinephrine, like many of the first-line agents today, may cause tremors, anxiety, and nausea, and most patients will tolerate these doses with no contraindications.[101] Even increased BP and tachycardia, which can also be attributed to severe anxiety, hypoxia, hypercapnia, and increased work of breathing, actually declined in the older cohort of patients, and only minimally increased in the younger group. In the younger group, BP and HR normalized when patients attained relief from bronchospasm.[101]

A second study published that same year was a study by Spiteri and colleagues[102] that compared terbutaline with epinephrine for the treatment of acute asthma, and it demonstrated that neither agent produced any significant increases in BP or HR, no treatment-related ECG abnormalities, and no observed adverse cardiovascular effects. Both of these studies showed benefit and no significant harm in the use of epinephrine for the treatment an asthmatic crisis. It is time to revisit this topic in a prospective and randomized manner.

Endotracheal Intubation

The decision to intubate should not be taken lightly as manipulation of the airway in a patient with AECOPD or an asthmatic crisis can cause laryngospasm, worsen bronchospasm, and may even increase morbidity. It is estimated that the mortality rate of ICU patients who are intubated for severe asthma is 10% to 20%.[103] Some studies have advocated that the severe asthmatic and COPD patient can be adequately managed without resorting to ETI.[104,105] Despite attempting to refrain from intubating a decompensating asthmatic, once first- and second-line therapies have failed, the practitioner must seriously consider ETI. The clinical decision regarding when to intubate a decompensating asthmatic patient can be aided by clinical signs such as an SaO_2 of less than 90% with maximal supplemental oxygen, bradypnea leading to hypercapnia and respiratory acidosis, altered level of consciousness, and physical exhaustion.[106] The only absolute indications for intubation are respiratory or cardiac arrest.[107]

The usual method for intubating a patient in AECOPD and asthmatic crisis is maximal preoxygenation followed by rapid sequence induction. Ketamine and propofol are both valid options for induction agents. Ketamine creates a catecholamine release that causes bronchodilation by relaxing bronchial smooth muscles.[108] Because this release of catecholamines can cause hypertension and arrhythmias, ketamine should be avoided in patients with active dysrhythmias. Propofol also has some bronchodilating effects, and it can cause hypotension. Patient selection for this drug also should be considered carefully.

Succinylcholine and rocuronium bromide are the 2 main choices of muscle relaxant for rapid sequence intubation in the ED. It is essential that their respective benefits and possible side effects be understood before selecting an agent. Traditionally, rocuronium has been considered to have a slower time of onset than succinylcholine. Importantly, onset is slower only if rocuronium is used at lower doses of 0.6 to 0.9 mg/kg IV. If a dose of 1.2 mg/kg IV is used, no difference exists in the time of onset of ideal intubating conditions, although the higher dose will lengthen the duration of paralysis.[109] The duration of paralysis with rocuronium is also dose dependent; time to paralysis recovery is reported to occur as early as 30 minutes with a dose of 0.6 mg/kg IV, and it will be double or even triple after a 1.2 mg/kg dose.[109] **Table 1** provides the common side effects encountered with succinylcholine. The most troubling and rare, side effect of rocuronium is anaphylaxis. Regardless of the agent used for paralysis, understanding respective mechanisms of action and side effects is essential.

In the patient with severe asthma and COPD, ETI and positive-pressure ventilation may cause abrupt increases in intrathoracic pressure that in turn decrease venous return and therefore cardiac output. For this reason, time permitting, it is important to optimize the patient's preload before ETI is attempted. A preintubation fluid bolus (as well as use of the ventilator strategies described elsewhere in this article) may help to prevent or attenuate abrupt decreases in BP immediately after ETI.

Post Endotracheal Intubation Documentation

ED and critical care specialists should be diligent in documenting the intubation procedure. A detailed medical record will greatly aid the clinician who attempts extubation when the pathophysiologic state has been reversed. The physician should always document the Cormack–Lehane grading scale (**Fig. 4**), the laryngoscope blade used, any airway adjuvants used, the number of intubation attempts made, a description of any complications, and any confirmation modalities used in the airway management.

Table 1	
Side effects of succinylcholine	
Side Effect	**Remarks**
Bradycardia	Occurs especially in small children after repeat doses.
Hyperkalemia	May increase potassium ~0.4 mmol/L in normal patients, but may lead to life-threatening increases in amyotrophic lateral sclerosis, multiple sclerosis, muscular dystrophies, inherited myopathies, denervating injuries, burns, and crush injuries
Fasciculations	Increase: • Oxygen consumption that may cause myalgia • Intragastric pressure, likely by increasing lower esophageal sphincter tone • Intracranial pressure • Intraocular pressure
Malignant hyperthermia	Rare

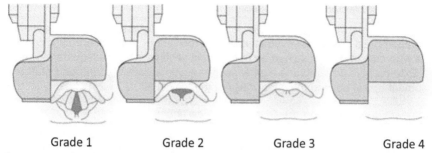

| Grade 1 | Grade 2 | Grade 3 | Grade 4 |

Fig. 4. Cormack–Lehane grading scale. (*From* Bjerkelund CE, Christensen P, Dragsund S, et al. [How to secure free airway?] Tidsskr Nor Laegeforen 2010;130(5):508; with permission.)

Delayed sequence intubation

Delayed sequence intubation (DSI) is an innovative technique used in a subset of the respiratory distress population that optimizes preoxygenation to achieve an oxygenation "safety net" before desaturation. This method allows for appropriate preoxygenation without the risk of gastric insufflation or aspiration.[110] As opposed to the traditional rapid sequence intubation method that consists of providing a sedative and paralytic agent simultaneously with no ventilation until ETI is attained,[111] DSI consists of providing a sedative agent that does not blunt the airway reflexes or spontaneous ventilation before administering the paralytic agent to place the endotracheal tube.[110] As mentioned, ketamine is considered by many as the optimal agent for DSI because it does not blunt patient airway reflexes or spontaneous respirations while providing a dissociative state that allows for the use of NIV,[112] and also providing the much warranted bronchodilation effects.[98–100] A second, and less efficacious agent that could be used, if ketamine's sympathomimetic effects are a concern, is dexmedetomidine, an α-2 agonist that provides sedation with no blunting of airway reflexes or respiratory drive.[113] Dexmedetomidine should not increase the patient's BP or HR; in fact, it can cause significant bradycardia. The typical initial bolus of this agent is 1 μg/kg over 10 minutes, and if needed, an infusion of 0.5 μg/kg per hour can be continued.[114,115] The final possible advantage that has been seen since the advent of DSI is that after the sedative agent and adequate NIV is provided to patients in respiratory failure, the respiratory state may improve in such a dramatic manner, that ETI may be avoided completely.[110] It is critical for providers to have adequate monitoring, time at the bedside, and ancillary support when attempting DSI.

Mechanical Ventilation

Once ETI is achieved, secured, and confirmed, the initial ventilator settings should be optimized to prevent hyperinflation and auto-PEEP in asthmatic and AECOPD patients. Hyperinflation pathophysiology could result in hypotension and barotrauma.[116] This goal is achieved by reducing both respiratory rate and tidal volume. These maneuvers shorten the inspiratory time and lengthen the time for exhalation, resulting in permissive hypercapnia. Permitting hypercapnia in this patient population is safer than causing hyperinflation while attempting to reach a normal $Paco_2$.[103] While intubated, the patient will require scheduled inhalational bronchodilator therapy to reverse the reactive airway disease process. Metered dose inhalers can be used instead of nebulizers, because they may decrease nosocomial pneumonia rates.[107] Deep sedation should be used in an attempt to minimize the use of neuromuscular blockade. Prolonged paralysis linked to neuromuscular blockade has been associated with increases in pneumonia rates and ICU duration of stay.[117]

Extracorporeal Membrane Oxygenation

The last resort in a clinically decompensating asthmatic patient would be the initiation of extracorporeal membrane oxygenation. This technology is considered in those patients who cannot be maintained on mechanical ventilation with adequate oxygenation. Extracorporeal membrane oxygenation requires a dedicated support staff and equipment and is beyond the capabilities of the typical ED.

Treatment Options Beyond the Emergency Department

The following therapies may also be used in the treatment of both severe asthmatic and COPD patients, but there is no evidence to support their use in the acute setting of the ED.

  i. Leukotriene modifiers
 ii. Mast cell stabilizers
iii. Anti-immunoglobulin therapy
 iv. Specific immunotherapy

MANAGEMENT BEYOND THE EMERGENCY DEPARTMENT

Weaning and extubation criteria have not been adequately studied in the acutely asthmatic or AECOPD patient.[103] AECOPD and asthma exacerbations that require ETI typically are slow to resolve and require aggressive therapy for more than 24 hours before weaning and extubation can be considered. Before assessing the patient for possible extubation, the practitioner must confirm that the asthmatic pathophysiologic state that warranted intubation has resolved. First, all sedation and muscle relaxants must be discontinued and prophylactic antiemetic treatment provided. The head of the bed should be raised to greater than 45°. Adequate time must be allowed for the patient to be able to follow simple commands, such as opening his eyes, tracking with his eyes, grasping with both hands, and protruding the tongue on command with no evidence of bronchospasm or hemodynamic compromise. Once appropriate time has elapsed, the cuff leak test should be performed. This test is used to evaluate for any laryngeal edema that might have occurred during the ETI and throughout the treatment. In the absence of laryngeal edema a noticeable airleak should be audible at the patient's bedside when the endotracheal tube cuff is deflated. Zhou and colleagues[118] state that the cuff test is accurate in finding significant differences in laryngeal edema, but that it does not accurately predict the need for reintubation. When no mucosal swelling is evident, the third step is the assessment of oxygenation and ventilation. Adequate oxygenation and ventilation can be assessed with a spontaneous breathing trial on reduced pressure support of 5 cm H_2O. If the patient is able to maintain the following parameters with no bronchospasm, an attempt at extubation can be considered[119]:

- SaO_2 of greater than 92% (PaO_2 >70) on FiO_2 less than 40% and PEEP is less than 5 cm H_2O;
- Tidal volume of greater than 5 mL/kg;
- Mean arterial pressure of greater than 60 with no aid of vasopressor agents;
- Respiratory rate of less than 30 and greater than 6 breaths/min; and
- HR of less than 100 and greater than 60 beats/min.

If the patient remains stable with no evidence of bronchospasm for approximately 30 minutes, one can move forward with the negative inspiratory force test. A value greater than −30 cm H_2O (normal, −90 to −120) indicates that the strength of the diaphragm and other inspiratory muscles is adequate to attempt extubation. A final assessment modality to predict a successful extubation is the rapid shallow breathing index. This index relies on the idea that patients on a ventilator who cannot tolerate independent breathing tend to breathe with high frequency and shallow tidal volume. Therefore, a score of less than approximately 100 is considered by most an adequate indication of weaning readiness.[120] Upon successful completion of all of these steps, extubation may be undertaken. Safe extubation of a patient requires equipment such as suction, oral airway, supplemental oxygen, and equipment that may be needed if reintubation is required. A nonrebreathing mask and NIV should be at the bedside because extubation may elicit laryngeal edema, bronchospasm, and postextubation stridor that require nebulized epinephrine and further treatment. In short, extubation should always be approached in a logical and cautious manner. Every step should be anticipated meticulously and executed cautiously to prevent reexacerbation or other complications.

ACUTE EXACERBATIONS OF CHRONIC OBSTRUCTIVE PULMONARY DISEASE AND ASTHMA CARE PLANS

The final component of post-AECOPD and asthmatic crisis care is a detailed COPD and asthma care plan that includes explicit discharge instructions, necessary medications and education in how to use them, education in self-assessment, a future action plan for managing recurrence of airflow obstruction, and an explicit follow-up appointment. COPD and asthma care plans, including education and case management, have been associated with improved outcomes and medication compliance. For the patient hospitalized with severe asthma or COPD, it is recommended that follow-up with an asthma/COPD-specialized clinician occur within 1 week of discharge. Pulmonary rehabilitation within the first 4 weeks after AECOPD is recommended to prevent acute exacerbations.[53] The final moments before the patient returns home after an asthmatic or AECOPD crisis are the ideal opportunity for clinicians to provide appropriate care plans that will assist patients with future exacerbations, encourage partnership with primary care physicians, and promote ongoing discussions of home asthma/COPD care.

REFERENCES

1. Moorman JE, Akinbami LJ, Bailey CM, et al. National surveillance of asthma: United States, 2001–2010. National Center for Health Statistics. Vital Health Stat 3 2012;(35):1–58. Available at: http://www.cdc.gov/nchs/data/series/sr_03/sr03_035.pdf.
2. Papaiwannou A, Zarogoulidis P, Porpodis K, et al. Asthma-chronic obstructive pulmonary disease overlap syndrome (ACOS): current literature review. J Thorac Dis 2014;6(Suppl 1):S146–51.
3. American Lung Association. Chronic obstructive pulmonary disease (COPD) fact sheet. Available at: http://www.lung.org/lung-disease/copd/resources/facts-figures/COPD-Fact-Sheet.html. Accessed November 24, 2014.
4. Global Initiative for Chronic Obstructive Lung Disease (GOLD). Global strategy for the diagnosis, management, and prevention of chronic obstructive pulmonary disease. 2013. Available at: http://www.goldcopd.org. Accessed January, 2015.
5. CDC's Asthma's Impact on the Nation. Available at: http://www.cdc.gov/asthma/most_recent_data.htm. Accessed January, 2015.

6. Ford ES. Hospital discharges, readmissions, and ED visits for COPD or bronchi-ectasis among US adults: findings from the Nationwide Inpatient Sample 2001-2012 and Nationwide Emergency Department Sample 2006-2011. Chest 2015;147(4):989–98.

7. Postma DS, Reddel HK, ten Hacken NH, et al. Asthma and chronic obstructive pulmonary disease: similarities and differences. Clin Chest Med 2014;35(1):143–56.

8. Global Initiative for Asthma (GINA). Global strategies for asthma management and prevention. 2015. Available at: www.ginasthma.org. Accessed January, 2015.

9. Sellers WFS. Inhaled and intravenous treatment in acute severe and life-threatening asthma. Br J Anaesth 2013;110(2):183–90.

10. Murata A, Ling PM. Asthma diagnosis and management. Emerg Med Clin North Am 2012;30:203–22.

11. National Asthma Education and Prevention Program. Expert panel report III: guidelines for the diagnosis and management of asthma. Bethesda (MD): National Heart, Lung, and Blood Institute; 2007. Available at: http://www.columbia.edu/cgi-bin/cul/resolve?clio7740011.

12. Fisher KA, Stefan MS, Darling C, et al. Impact of COPD on the mortality and treatment of patients hospitalized with acute decompensated heart failure: the Worcester Heart Failure Study. Chest 2015;147(3):637–45.

13. De Blois J, Simard S, Atar D, et al. COPD predicts mortality in HF: the Norwegian Heart Failure Registry. J Card Fail 2010;16(3):225–9.

14. Macchia A, Monte S, Romero M, et al. The prognostic influence of chronic obstructive pulmonary disease in patients hospitalised for chronic heart failure. Eur J Heart Fail 2007;9(9):942–8.

15. Mohan A, Chandra S, Agarwal D, et al. Prevalence of viral infection detected by PCR and RT-PCR in patients with acute exacerbation of COPD: a systematic review. Respirology 2010;15(3):536–42.

16. Kelly AM. Agreement between arterial and venous blood gases in emergency medical care: a systematic review Hong Kong. J Emerg Med 2013;20:166–71.

17. Kelly AM, Kerr D, Middleton P. Validation of venous pCO2 to screen for arterial hypercarbia in patients with chronic obstructive airways disease. J Emerg Med 2005;28:377–9.

18. Kelly AM, Kyle E, McAlpine R. Venous pCO2 and pH can be used to screen for significant hypercarbia in emergency patients with acute respiratory disease. J Emerg Med 2002;22:15–9.

19. Sur E. COPD: is it all in the vein? Thorax 2013;68(Suppl 3):P182.

20. McCanny P, Bennett K, Staunton P, et al. Venous vs. arterial blood gases in the assessment of patients presenting with an exacerbation of chronic obstructive pulmonary disease. Am J Emerg Med 2012;30:896–900.

21. Ibrahim I, Ooi SBS, Huak CY, et al. Point-of-care bedside gas analyzer: limited use of venous pCO2 in emergency patients. J Emerg Med 2011;41:117–23.

22. Lim BL, Kelly AM. A meta-analysis on the utility of peripheral venous blood gas analysis in exacerbations of chronic obstructive pulmonary disease in the emergency department. Eur J Emerg Med 2010;17:246–8.

23. Razi E, Moosavi GA. Comparison of arterial and venous blood gases analysis in patients with exacerbation of chronic obstructive pulmonary disease. Saudi Med J 2007;28:862–5.

24. Ak A, Ogun CO, Bayor A, et al. Prediction of arterial blood gas values from venous blood gas values in patients with acute exacerbation of chronic obstructive pulmonary disease. Tohoku J Exp Med 2006;210:285–90.

25. Rang LCF, Murray HE, Wells GA, et al. Can peripheral venous blood gases replace arterial blood gases in emergency department patients? CJEM 2002;4:7–15.

26. Elborn JS, Finch MB, Stanford CF. Non-arterial assessment of blood gas status in patients with chronic pulmonary disease. Ulster Med J 1991;60:164–7.

27. Doğan NÖ, Şener A, Günaydın GP, et al. The accuracy of mainstream end-tidal carbon dioxide levels to predict the severity of chronic obstructive pulmonary disease exacerbations presented to the ED. Am J Emerg Med 2014;32(5): 408–11.

28. Cinar O, Acar YA, Arziman I, et al. Can mainstream end-tidal carbon dioxide measurement accurately predict the arterial carbon dioxide level of patients with acute dyspnea in ED. Am J Emerg Med 2012;30:358–61.

29. Murray CJ, Atkinson C, Bhalla K, et al. The State of US health, 1990-2010: burden of diseases, injuries, and risk factors. JAMA 2013;310:591–608.

30. Curkendall SM, DeLuise C, Jones JK, et al. Cardiovascular disease in patients with chronic obstructive pulmonary disease, Saskatchewan Canada cardiovascular disease in COPD patients. Ann Epidemiol 2006;16:63–70.

31. Schneider C, Bothner U, Jick SS, et al. Chronic obstructive pulmonary disease and the risk of cardiovascular diseases. Eur J Epidemiol 2010;25:253–60.

32. Shah NS, Koller SM, Janower ML, et al. Diaphragm levels as determinants of P axis in restrictive vs obstructive pulmonary disease. Chest 1995;107(3): 697–700.

33. Rodman DM, Lowenstein SR, Rodman T. The electrocardiogram in chronic obstructive pulmonary disease. J Emerg Med 1990;8:607–15.

34. Thomas AJ, Apiyasawat S, Spodick DH. Electrocardiographic detection of emphysema. Am J Cardiol 2011;107:1090–2.

35. Khalid N, Chhabra L, Spodick DH. Electrocardiographic screening of emphysema: lead aVL or Leads III and I? Acta Inform Med 2013;21(3):223.

36. Friedman PJ. Imaging studies in emphysema. Proc Am Thorac Soc 2008;5: 494–500.

37. Tsai T, Gallagher E, Lombardi G, et al. Guidelines for the selective ordering of admission chest radiography in adult obstructive airway disease. Ann Emerg Med 1993;22:1854–8.

38. Rizkallah J, Man SF, Sin DD. Prevalence of pulmonary embolism in acute exacerbations of COPD: a systematic review and metaanalysis. Chest 2009;135: 786–93.

39. Lichtenstein D, van Hooland S, Elbers P, et al. Ten good reasons to practice ultrasound in critical care. Anaesthesiol Intensive Ther 2014;46(5):323–35.

40. Gallard E, Redonnet JP, Bourcier JE, et al. Diagnostic performance of cardiopulmonary ultrasound performed by the emergency physician in the management of acute dyspnea. Am J Emerg Med 2015;33(3):352–8.

41. Silva S, Biendel C, Ruiz J, et al. Usefulness of cardiothoracic chest ultrasound in the management of acute respiratory failure in critical care practice. Chest 2013; 144(3):859–65.

42. Sassoon CSH, Hassell KT, Mahutte CK. Hypoxic induced hypercapnia in stable chronic obstructive pulmonary disease. Am Rev Respir Dis 1987;135:907–11.

43. Susanto C, Thomas PS. Assessing the use of initial oxygen therapy in chronic obstructive pulmonary disease patients: a retrospective audit of pre-hospital and hospital emergency management. Intern Med J 2015;45(5):510–6.

44. Austin M, Wills E, Blizzard L, et al. Effect of high flow oxygen on mortality on chronic obstructive pulmonary disease patients in prehospital setting: randomised controlled trial. BMJ 2010;341:c546.

45. Beasley R, Aldington S, Robinson G. Is it time to change the approach to oxygen therapy in the breathless patient? Thorax 2007;62:840–1.
46. Ameredes BT, Calhoun WJ. Albuterol enantiomers: pre-clinical and clinical value? Front Biosci (Elite Ed) 2010;2:1081–92.
47. Andrews T, McGintee E, Mittal MK, et al. High-dose continuous nebulized levalbuterol for pediatric status asthmaticus: a randomized trial. J Pediatr 2009;155: 205–10.
48. Wilkinson M, Bulloch B, Garcia-Filion P, et al. Efficacy of racemic albuterol versus levalbuterol used as a continuous nebulization for the treatment of acute asthma exacerbations: a randomized, double-blind, clinical trial. J Asthma 2011;48(2):188–93.
49. Jat KR, Khairwa A. Levalbuterol versus albuterol for acute asthma: A systematic review and meta-analysis. Pulm Pharmacol Ther 2013;26(2):239–48.
50. Castle W, Fuller R, Hall J, et al. Serevent nationwide surveillance study: comparison of salmeterol with salbutamol in asthmatic patients who require regular bronchodilator treatment. BMJ 1993;306:1034–7.
51. Nelson HS, Weiss ST, Bleecker ER, et al. The salmeterol multicenter asthma research trial: a comparison of usual pharmacotherapy for asthma or usual pharmacotherapy plus salmeterol. Chest 2006;129:15–26.
52. Mann M, Chowdhury B, Sullivan E, et al. Serious asthma exacerbations in asthmatics treated with high-dose formoterol. Chest 2003;124:70–4.
53. Criner GL, Bourbeau J, Diekemper RL, et al. Prevention of Acute Exacerbations of COPD: American College of Chest Physicians and Canadian Thoracic Society Guideline. Chest 2015;147(4):894–942.
54. Rennard SI. Treatment of stable chronic obstructive pulmonary disease. Lancet 2004;364(9436):791–802.
55. Vézina K, Chauhan BF, Ducharme FM. Inhaled anticholinergics and short-acting beta(2)-agonists versus short-acting beta2-agonists alone for children with acute asthma in hospital. Cochrane Database Syst Rev 2014;(7):CD010283.
56. Rodrigo GJ, Castro-Rodriguez JA. Anticholinergics in the treatment of children and adults with acute asthma: a systematic review with meta-analysis. Thorax 2005;60:740–6.
57. Plotnick LH, Ducharme FM. Acute asthma in children and adolescents: should inhaled anticholinergics be added to beta(2)-agonists? Am J Respir Med 2003;2:109–15.
58. Zorc JJ, Pusic MV, Ogborn CJ, et al. Ipratropium bromide added to asthma treatment in the pediatric emergency department. Pediatrics 1999;103(4 Pt 1):748–52.
59. Kerstjens HA, Engel M, Dahl R, et al. Tiotropium in asthma poorly controlled with standard combination therapy. N Engl J Med 2012;367:1198–207.
60. Teoh L, Cates CJ, Hurwitz M, et al. Anticholinergic therapy for acute asthma in children. Cochrane Database Syst Rev 2012;(4):CD003797.
61. Craven D, Kercsmar CM, Myers TR, et al. Ipratropium bromide plus nebulized albuterol for the treatment of hospitalized children with acute asthma. J Pediatr 2001;138(1):51–8.
62. Goggin N, Macarthur C, Parkin PC. Randomized trial of the addition of ipratropium bromide to albuterol and corticosteroid therapy in children hospitalized because of an acute asthma exacerbation. Arch Pediatr Adolesc Med 2001; 155(12):1329–34.
63. Cates CJ, Crilly JA, Rowe BH. Holding chambers (spacers) versus nebulisers for beta-agonist treatment of acute asthma. Cochrane Database Syst Rev 2006;(2):CD000052.

64. Turner MO, Gafni A, Swan D, et al. A review and economic evaluation of bronchodilator delivery methods in hospitalized patients. Arch Intern Med 1996;156: 2113–8.
65. Rodrigo GL. Advances in acute asthma. Curr Opin Pulm Med 2015;21(1):22–6.
66. Goodacre S, Cohen J, Bradburn M, et al. Intravenous or nebulised magnesium sulphate versus standard therapy for severe acute asthma (3Mg trial): a double-blind, randomised controlled trial. Lancet Respir Med 2013;1:293–300.
67. Kew KM, Kirtchuk L, Michell CI. Intravenous magnesium sulfate for treating adults with acute asthma in the emergency department. Cochrane Database Syst Rev 2014;(5):CD010909.
68. Walters JA, Tan DJ, White CJ, et al. Systemic corticosteroids for acute exacerbations of chronic obstructive pulmonary disease. Cochrane Database Syst Rev 2014;(9):CD001288.
69. Kiser TH, Vandivier RW. Severe acute exacerbations of chronic obstructive pulmonary disease: does the dosage of corticosteroids and type of antibiotic matter? Curr Opin Pulm Med 2015;21:142–8.
70. Lindenauer PK, Pekow PS, Lahti MC, et al. Association of corticosteroid dose and route of administration with risk of treatment failure in acute exacerbation of chronic obstructive pulmonary disease. JAMA 2010;303:2359–67.
71. Mendes ES, Cadet L, Arana J, et al. Acute effect of an inhaled glucocorticosteroid on albuterol-induced bronchodilation in patients with moderately severe asthma. Chest 2015;147(4):1037–42.
72. Cheng T, Gong Y, Guo Y, et al. Systemic corticosteroid for COPD exacerbations, whether the higher dose is better? A meta-analysis of randomized controlled trials. Clin Respir J 2013;7:305–18.
73. Alia I, de la Cal MA, Esteban A, et al. Efficacy of corticosteroid therapy in patients with an acute exacerbation of chronic obstructive pulmonary disease receiving ventilatory support. Arch Intern Med 2011;171:1939–46.
74. Schacke H, Schottelius A, Docke WD, et al. Dissociation of transactivation from transrepression by a selective glucocorticoid receptor agonist leads to separation of therapeutic effects from side effects. Proc Natl Acad Sci U S A 2004;101:227–32.
75. Schacke H, Docke WD, Asadullah K. Mechanisms involved in the side effects of glucocorticoids. Pharmacol Ther 2002;96:23–43.
76. Kiser TH, Allen RR, Valuck RJ, et al. Outcomes associated with corticosteroid dosage in critically ill patients with acute exacerbations of chronic obstructive pulmonary disease. Am J Respir Crit Care Med 2014;189:1052–64.
77. Leuppi JD, Schuetz P, Bingisser R, et al. Short-term vs conventional glucocorticoid therapy in acute exacerbations of chronic obstructive pulmonary disease: the REDUCE randomized clinical trial. JAMA 2013;309:2223–31.
78. Available at: http://emupdates.com/2011/12/14/when-the-patient-cant-breathe-and-you-cant-think-the-emergency-departement-life-threatening-asthma-flowsheet/. Accessed January, 2015.
79. Domenech A, Puig C, Marti S, et al. Infectious etiology of acute exacerbations in severe COPD patients. J Infect 2013;67:516–23.
80. Decramer M, Janssens W, Miravitlles M. Chronic obstructive pulmonary disease. Lancet 2012;379:1341–51.
81. Sethi S, Murphy TF. Infection in the pathogenesis and course of chronic obstructive pulmonary disease. N Engl J Med 2008;359:2355–65.
82. White AJ, Gompertz S, Bayley DL, et al. Resolution of bronchial inflammation is related to bacterial eradication following treatment of exacerbations of chronic bronchitis. Thorax 2003;58:680–5.

83. Martinez FJ, Curtis JL, Albert R. Role of macrolide therapy in chronic obstructive pulmonary disease. Int J Chron Obstruct Pulmon Dis 2008;3:331–50.
84. Barnes PJ. Corticosteroid resistance in patients with asthma and chronic obstructive pulmonary disease. J Allergy Clin Immunol 2013;131:636–45.
85. Carson KV, Usmani ZA, Smith BJ. Noninvasive ventilation in acute severe asthma: current evidence and future perspectives. Curr Opin Pulm Med 2014; 20:118–23.
86. Buda AJ, Pinsky MR, Ingels NB Jr, et al. Effect of intrathoracic pressure on left ventricular performance. N Engl J Med 1979;301:453–9.
87. Broux R, Foidart G, Mendes P, et al. Use of PEEP in management of life- threatening status asthmaticus: a method for the recovery of appropriate ventilation-perfusion ratio. Appl Cardiopulm Pathophysiol 1991;4:79–83.
88. Soroksky S, Stav D, Shpirer I. A pilot prospective, randomized, placebo-controlled trial of bilevel positive airway pressure in acute asthmatic attack. Chest 2003;123:1018–25.
89. Nourdine K, Combes P, Carton MJ, et al. Does noninvasive ventilation reduce the ICU nosocomial infection risk? A prospective clinical survey. Intensive Care Med 1999;25:567–73.
90. Lim WJ, Mohammed Akram R, Carson KV, et al. Noninvasive positive & pressure ventilation for treatment of respiratory failure due to severe acute exacerbations of asthma. Cochrane Database Syst Rev 2012;(12):CD004360.
91. Yeow ME, Santanilla JI. Noninvasive positive pressure ventilation in the emergency department. Emerg Med Clin North Am 2008;26:835–47.
92. Nishimura M. High-flow nasal cannula oxygen therapy in adults. J Intensive Care 2015;3:15.
93. Corley A, Caruana LR, Barnett AG, et al. Oxygen delivery through high-flow nasal cannulae increase end-expiratory lung volume and reduce respiratory rate in post-cardiac surgical patients. Br J Anaesth 2011;107(6):998–1004.
94. El-Khatib MF, Jamaleddine G. Effect of heliox- and air-driven nebulized bronchodilator therapy on lung function in patients with asthma. Lung 2014;192:377–83.
95. Bag R, Bandi V, Fromm RE Jr, et al. The effect of heliox-driven bronchodilator aerosol therapy on pulmonary function tests in patients with asthma. J Asthma 2002;39(7):659–65.
96. Rodrigo GJ, Rodriguez-Castro JA. Heliox-driven β2-agonists nebulization for children and adults with acute asthma: a systematic review with meta-analysis. Ann Allergy Asthma Immunol 2014;112:29–34.
97. Stevenson C. Ketamine: a review. Update Anaesth 2005;20:25–9.
98. Sato T, Hirota K, Matsuki A, et al. The role of the N-Methyl-D-Aspartic acid receptor in the relaxant effect of ketamine on tracheal smooth muscle. Anesth Analg 1998;87:1383–8.
99. Zhu MM, Qian YN, Zhu W, et al. Protective effects of ketamine on allergen-induced airway inflammatory injure and high airway reactivity in asthma: experiment with rats. Zhonghua Yi Xue Za Zhi 2007;87:1308–13.
100. Goyal S, Agrawal A. Ketamine in status asthmaticus: a review. Indian J Crit Care Med 2013;17(3):154–61.
101. Cydulka R, Davison R, Grammer L, et al. The use of epinephrine in the treatment of older adult asthmatics. Ann Emerg Med 1988;17(4):322–6.
102. Spiteri MA, Millar AB, Pavia D, et al. Subcutaneous adrenaline versus terbutaline for the treatment of acute severe asthma. Thorax 1988;43(1):19–23.
103. Brenner B, Corbridge T, Kazzi A. Intubation and mechanical ventilation of the patient in respiratory failure. J Emerg Med 2009;37(2S):S23–34.

104. Braman SS, Kaemmerlen JT. Intensive care of status asthmaticus. A 10-year experience. JAMA 1990;264:366–8.
105. Mountain RD, Sahn SA. Acid-base disturbances in acute asthma. Chest 1990; 98:651–5.
106. Murase K, Tomii K, Chin K, et al. The use of non-invasive ventilation for life-threatening asthma attacks: changes in the need for intubation. Respirology 2010;15:714–20.
107. Schauer SG, Cuenca PJ, Johnson JJ, et al. Management of acute asthma in the emergency department. Emerg Med Pract 2013;15(6):1–28.
108. Brown RH, Wagner EM. Mechanisms of bronchoprotection by anesthetic induction agents: propofol versus ketamine. Anesthesiology 1999;90:822–8.
109. Perry JJ, Lee JS, Sillberg VA, et al. Rocuronium versus succinylcholine for rapid sequence induction intubation. Cochrane Database Syst Rev 2008;(2):CD002788.
110. Weingart SD. Preoxygenation, reoxygenation, and delayed sequence intubation in the emergency department. J Emerg Med 2011;40(6):661–7.
111. Walls RM, Murphy MF. Manual of emergency airway management. 3rd edition. Philadelphia: Lippincott Williams & Wilkins; 2008.
112. Aroni F, Iacovidou N, Dontas I, et al. Pharmacological aspects and potential new clinical applications of ketamine: reevaluation of an old drug. J Clin Pharmacol 2009;49:957–64.
113. Carollo DS, Nossaman BD, Ramadhyani U. Dexmedetomidine: a review of clinical applications. Curr Opin Anaesthesiol 2008;21:457–61.
114. Abdelmalak B, Makary L, Hoban J, et al. Dexmedetomidine as sole sedative for awake intubation in management of the critical airway. J Clin Anesth 2007;19: 370–3.
115. Bergese SD, Khabiri B, Roberts WD, et al. Dexmedetomidine for conscious sedation in difficult awake fiberoptic intubation cases. J Clin Anesth 2007;19: 141–4.
116. Lougheed MD, Fisher T, O'Donnell DE. Dynamic hyperinflation during bronchoconstriction in asthma: implications for symptom perception. Chest 2006;130: 1072–81.
117. Adnet F, Racine SX, Lapostolle F, et al. Full reversal of hypercapnic coma by noninvasive positive pressure ventilation. Am J Emerg Med 2001;19:244–6.
118. Zhou T, Zhang HP, Chen WW, et al. Cuff-leak test for predicting postextubation airway complications: a systematic review. J Evid Based Med 2011;4(4):242–54.
119. Salam A, Tilluckdharry L, Amoateng-Adjepong Y, et al. Neurologic status, cough, secretions and extubation outcomes. Intensive Care Med 2004;30: 1334–9.
120. Meade M, Guyatt G, Cook D, et al. Predicting success in weaning from mechanical ventilation. Chest 2001;120(6 Suppl):400S–24S.

Respiratory Emergencies in Geriatric Patients

Katren Tyler, MD*, Dane Stevenson, MD

KEYWORDS

- Acute dyspnea • Respiratory emergency • Lungs • Geriatric

KEY POINTS

- Almost every disease process that primarily affects the lung is more common in older patients.
- Even in healthy older adults, there are significant age-related lung changes.
- Influenza is estimated to cause 35,000 deaths annually in older patients in the United States.
- Chronic obstructive pulmonary disease (COPD) accounts for nearly 20% of all hospital admissions in people 65 to 75 years old.
- Short courses of antibiotics are as effective as longer courses for acute exacerbations of COPD.
- Age-adjusted D-dimer values have been validated and are likely to be increasingly incorporated into clinical decision rules.
- Emergency departments are the first entry into the health care system for 80% of patients with acute heart failure.
- Noninvasive ventilation should be used early and liberally for patients with acute respiratory failure.

RESPIRATORY EMERGENCIES IN GERIATRIC PATIENTS

In the United States, patients more than 65 years old currently account for 13% of the population and this number is anticipated to increase to 20% by 2030.[1] In 2020 the number of people more than the age of 65 years will exceed those less than 5 years old worldwide for the first time in history.[2] The population pyramid has become a rectangle.

Almost every disease process that primarily affects the lung is more common in older patients. Many lung diseases are more common in older patients or are seen almost exclusively in older patients.[3] Pulmonary disease in an older person increases the likelihood of developing geriatric syndromes like recurrent falls and frailty.[4]

Disclosures: The authors have no financial disclosures or conflicts of interest.
Department of Emergency Medicine, University of California, Davis, 4150 V Street, PSSB 2100, Sacramento, CA 95817, USA
* Corresponding author.
E-mail address: krtyler@ucdavis.edu

Emerg Med Clin N Am 34 (2016) 39–49
http://dx.doi.org/10.1016/j.emc.2015.08.003
emed.theclinics.com

Older patients typically have more than one disease process. Clinical studies often exclude older patients, and clinical studies often exclude patients with multiple morbidities. Published studies may have limited applicability to complex older patients with multiple morbidities. In addition to their multiple morbidities, older patients are more likely to have cognitive impairment and medication adherence issues, and to require caregiver involvement, and are more likely to live in an institution.[4] Focusing clinical attention on a single disease process in an older patient might negatively affect the management of other conditions and thus the patient as a whole.[5]

Clinically, distinguishing the cause of acute dyspnea in the emergency department can be challenging in older adults with multiple morbidities. Management and evaluation of acute dyspnea remains one of the key skills of emergency medicine because they must take place simultaneously, and treatment must be initiated before any diagnostic studies have returned.

AGE-RELATED LUNG CHANGES

Even in healthy older adults, there are significant age-related lung changes. These age-related lung changes result in a reduced pulmonary reserve when faced with an acute disease process. Older patients are more susceptible to viral and bacterial pneumonias, and are more likely to experience a more severe clinical course. Older patients are at increased risk of adult respiratory distress syndrome, venous thromboembolism, and late-onset asthma associated with lung remodeling.[3,6]

Older patients experience age-related physiologic changes in chest wall stiffness, elastic lung recoil, and in respiratory muscle strength.[4] Increasing kyphosis secondary to loss of height of intervertebral discs makes the lung cavity smaller because of a narrowing of the rib spaces. Kyphosis increases from age 40 years, and is seen more commonly in women. Normal thoracic kyphosis is under 40°; however, once kyphosis exceeds 55° there are significant reductions in forced expiratory volume (FEV) and forced vital capacity (FVC). An effective cough requires the ability to generate a large inspiratory volume. The overall effectiveness of the mucociliary elevator that removes small and large particles is reduced by aging and significantly affected by smoking. Aging is also associated with complex changes in immunity.[6] In addition to the role of cognitive impairment in taking a history, both cognitive impairment and sarcopenia may interfere with the ability to perform spirometry and to self-administer inhaled medications.[4]

Older people are increasingly obese in both developed and developing countries and the pulmonary consequences of obesity extend beyond simple mechanics and physiology. By 2030, approximately 50% of the US population is projected to have a body mass index greater than 30, of whom 24 million people will be older than age 60 years.[7] From a respiratory perspective, obese patients are at risk of developing late-onset asthma, pulmonary hypertension, acute lung injury, and complications of lung infections.[8–10]

RESPIRATORY INFECTIONS: VIRAL

Influenza is estimated to cause 35,000 deaths annually in older patients in the United States[11] and influenza and influenza-like illnesses have a high morbidity in older patients. During the 2014 to 2015 influenza season, the rates of hospitalization for laboratory-confirmed influenza in the United States were 258 per 100,000 population for patients more than 65 years old, compared with 41 per 100,000 population for patients 50 to 64 years old.[12] More than 90% of deaths attributable to influenza occur in patients more than 65 years old,[13] and, during influenza epidemics, combined pneumonia and influenza deaths account for up to 10% of all mortality throughout the population.[12]

Excellent supportive care remains the foundation of management of all patients with influenza, including the elderly. Fluid management, high-calorie nutrition, antipyretics for comfort, and encouragement of mobility are important. Vigilance for the complications of influenza, particularly pneumonia, delirium, pressure areas, and sepsis, is critical. Antiviral drugs can be used to treat influenza and as an adjunct to immunization for postexposure prophylaxis in high-risk individuals. Three antiviral agents are effective against both influenza A and B. Oseltamivir (Tamiflu) is taken orally, and zanamivir (Relenza) is inhaled. Peramivir is a newer agent available only in an intravenous formulation. Antiviral agents can reduce both the severity and the duration of influenza, are usually well tolerated, but should be taken within 48 hours of symptom onset for maximal benefit.[14] Antiviral therapy against influenza is recommended for patients who are at high risk of complications, including children less than 2 years old, adults more than 65 years old, the morbidly obese, and pregnant patients.[14]

Influenza spreads by respiratory droplets. In addition to the risk of contracting influenza in the community, older patients are particularly at risk of contracting influenza from health care workers (HCW) infected with influenza or from other infected patients in the emergency department. HCW are also at risk of contracting influenza from their patients. Droplet-generating procedures include nebulized breathing treatments, intubation, and mechanical ventilation, including noninvasive ventilation (NIV). Viral shedding of influenza virus lasts at least 5 days, including 24 hours before the development of fever, and perhaps longer in critically ill patients.[13] Encouraging vaccination of HCW through voluntary or mandatory procedures limits spread within institutions.[15] The effectiveness of the vaccination year to year depends on the dominant viral strains. Other behaviors within the health care system that limit the spread of influenza include cohorting infected patients, limiting patient movements between departments, the use of face masks, and asking infected visitors and HCW to stay home. HCW should stay home until they have not had a fever for 48 hours.

Bacterial Pneumonia

Pneumonia is an acute respiratory inflammation usually caused by a viral or bacterial infection associated with radiographic shadowing on a chest radiograph. Pneumonia is also seen occasionally in response to chemical irritation, such as aspiration pneumonia. The pathogens responsible for the development of pneumonia differ depending on where the patient resides.

Older patients who live independently at home are at risk for the typical bacterial pneumonias, such as *Streptococcus pneumoniae*, *Haemophilus influenzae*, and less commonly gram-negative bacilli, and the atypical organisms *Legionella pneumophila*, and *Mycoplasma pneumoniae*. Even in older community-dwelling adults, viral pneumonia is the second most common cause of community-acquired pneumonia (CAP). Coverage for CAP is directed at both the typical and atypical organisms but does not usually include coverage against *Staphylococcus aureus*.

Patients residing within a skilled nursing facility are also at risk of the standard viral and bacterial pathogens, but have an increased risk from gram-negative bacilli such as *Klebsiella* and *Pseudomonas aeruginosa*, and from anaerobes such as *Bacteroides*, especially in frail and immobile patients with a risk of aspiration. Antibiotic treatment of health care–associated pneumonia broadens the spectrum to include coverage for anaerobes and gram-negative bacilli, especially *P aeruginosa*.

Following influenza infections, patients are at risk of secondary bacterial infection from *S pneumoniae*, *H influenzae*, or *S aureus*.

Frail older patients may not present with the typical fever, cough, and shortness of breath that characterizes younger patients with pneumonia. Many older patients with pneumonia present with a cough (often nonproductive), delirium, anorexia, falls and dizziness, or may present with signs of severe sepsis. Older patients who present with hypothermia and sepsis from pneumonia have significant in-hospital mortality.[16]

Pneumonia scoring systems to evaluate the safety of outpatient management, such as the CURB-65 (confusion, increased urea level, respiratory rate, blood pressure, and age>65 years) and the Pneumonia Severity Index, all include age as one of the primary variables, with age greater than 70 years automatically being associated with a higher risk.[17]

Treatment of pneumonia is directed at general supportive care with targeted antibiotic therapy, often initially broad-spectrum therapy. Oxygen should be provided to keep arterial oxygen saturation (SaO_2) greater than 92% and fluid balance optimized. Mobility should be encouraged, venous thromboembolism prophylaxis commenced, and oral intake encouraged as long as the aspiration risk is minimized. The adage of the anticipated clinical course can be useful in discussing the prognosis with the patient and the family, and planning ahead for possible deterioration is wise. If the older patient has already made choices regarding life-sustaining treatments, such as Physician Orders for Life-sustaining Treatments, this is an excellent opportunity to review these plans and goals for care.

CHRONIC OBSTRUCTIVE PULMONARY DISEASE

Chronic obstructive pulmonary disease (COPD) has become the fourth leading cause of death worldwide and the third leading cause of death in the United States.[18] The prevalence of COPD in people more than 65 years old is 10% to 14% regardless of exposure, and COPD accounts for nearly 20% of all hospital admissions in people 65 to 75 years.[19] Most of the mortality in COPD occurs in patients more than 65 years of age.

The primary symptoms of COPD are chronic cough, chronic sputum production, and dyspnea. The major risk factor in developed countries is exposure to tobacco smoke. Assessment of COPD is based on the patient's symptoms, spirometry, risk of exacerbations, and the identification of comorbidities. There is no cure for COPD and there are no disease-modifying agents for COPD. The use of pharmacology, smoking cessation, and pulmonary rehabilitation can reduce symptoms and the frequency and severity of acute exacerbations, improve health status, and improve exercise tolerance. A COPD exacerbation is an acute event of deteriorating respiratory symptoms beyond the normal daily variability,[20] but, it is not always clear whether symptoms represent a new deterioration.

Spirometry is required to make a clinical diagnosis of COPD; the presence of a post-bronchodilator FEV in 1 second (FEV1)/FVC less than 0.70 confirms the presence of persistent airflow limitation and thus of COPD. The Global Initiative for Chronic Obstructive Lung Disease (GOLD) criteria use 4 stages based on both spirometry measurements and symptoms, with stage IV being the most severe (FEV1<30% predicted with chronic respiratory failure). Basing the diagnosis of COPD only on spirometry leads to overdiagnosis of COPD in older patients because of the normal aging of the lung.[4,18,21]

The differential diagnosis of COPD includes asthma with reversible airflow limitation, congestive heart failure (HF) with cardiac wheeze caused by narrowing of the bronchioles from pulmonary edema, bronchiectasis characterized by copious sputum, recurrent aspiration, vocal cord dysfunction, and angiotensin-converting enzyme inhibitor–induced cough (this may have normal spirometry).[4,20,21]

Management of COPD includes pharmacologic and nonpharmacologic interventions. Pharmacologic interventions include a stepwise progression with a short-acting bronchodilator (mostly beta-2 agonists) on an as-needed basis, then regular treatment in addition to as needed, then add a long-acting bronchodilator, an inhaled corticosteroid, and also a combination long-acting agent (long-acting beta-2 agonist plus long-acting anticholinergic). After these measures, consider long-term oxygen and noninvasive positive pressure ventilation (NPPV).[4,18,20–23] Systemic anticholinergic effects from inhaled anticholinergics such as ipratropium or tiotropium are not seen in older patients. Inhaled medications depend on drug delivery to the lungs, and the use of inhaled medication devices may be compromised by arthritis, loss of muscle strength, cognitive impairment, and vision loss.[4,18,20–23]

Nonpharmacologic measures in the management of COPD include smoking cessation, pulmonary rehabilitation, osteoporosis evaluation, and vaccinations against influenza and pneumococcus. Older patients with COPD are likely to benefit from frequent reevaluations of goals of care, reinforcement of proper inhaler technique, and screening for depression and anxiety.[4,20] Smoking cessation remains a critical event in patients with COPD. Older patients are less likely than younger patients to be encouraged to stop smoking by hospital physicians. Medications used to assist in smoking cessation, such as bupropion, may have significant neuropsychiatric effects in older patients.[4]

All patients with COPD with breathlessness, when walking at their own pace on level ground, seem to benefit from rehabilitation and maintenance of physical activity.[20] Patients with COPD should be encouraged to maintain their physical activity, because an increasingly sedentary lifestyle results in a negative cycle of worsening dyspnea with activity and deconditioning.[4,20] The role of emergency physicians in encouraging formal pulmonary rehabilitation and informal physical activity has not been explored.

ACUTE EXACERBATIONS OF CHRONIC OBSTRUCTIVE PULMONARY DISEASE

About 70% of acute exacerbations of COPD (AECOPD) are caused by viral or bacterial infections.[4,19,20] Many patients with COPD have significant bacterial colonization at baseline but sputum isolated during AECOPD seems to be associated with new strains. Evidence supports antibiotic use for patients with severe COPD and 2 of the following symptoms: increased dyspnea, sputum purulence, and increased sputum volume. Antibiotic coverage should be broadened to include pseudomonal coverage in patients with moderate to severe COPD, a history of recurrent hospitalizations, or known or suspected underlying bronchiectasis with copious sputum production.[4,19] Treatment duration has been questioned recently with short courses (<5 days) having been shown to be as effective as longer courses (>5 days).[24]

Corticosteroids for AECOPD are recommended, given orally at 30 to 40 mg unless oral use is contraindicated. There are suggestions that the duration of therapy might need to be 7 to 10 days, with maximal benefits of steroids not seen until 5 days.[4]

NIV can be of significant value in AECOPD, and is appropriately used as a first-line treatment in many emergency departments.[25–28] Excluding the short-term use of NIV as a bridge to intubation, patients who are placed on NIV for AECOPD should be awake enough to maintain their own airway. Patients with copious amounts of secretion may not do well on NIV but warrant a short trial. Up to 30% of patients with AECOPD are not able to tolerate the NIV mask.[28]

PULMONARY EMBOLISM

Conditions predisposing to venous thromboembolism (VTE) occur commonly in older populations, and most pulmonary emboli (PEs) occur in older patients.[29] The incidence of VTE in older patients is more than 1% per year.[30] In particular, malignancy and postoperative states and resulting immobility are more common in older patients. The signs and symptoms of PE are not specific to the diagnosis and are easily confused with other symptoms in older patients with multimorbidity. Older patients with confirmed PE are less likely to have pleuritic chest pain and more likely to present with syncope than younger patients.[30]

Although the overall risk of VTE is increased in older patients, there is a proportionally larger age-related increase in D-dimer levels. Only 5% of patients more than 80 years old have a negative D-dimer, compared with 50% of patients less than 50 years old.[30] Clinical prediction rules that use D-dimer levels to exclude low-risk patients from needing further imaging studies are negatively affected by expected age-related increases in D-dimer levels.

Recent strategies for addressing the expected age-related increase in D-dimer levels have been published and significantly reduce the number of advanced imaging studies that are ordered without affecting morbidity or mortality. Age-adjusted D-dimer cutoffs have been validated for use in low-risk patients more than 50 years old (revised Geneva Score of "Not high" or Wells Score of "Low")[31,32] and are beginning to be incorporated into clinical decision tools.[33,34] The simplest form uses an age-adjusted D-dimer cutoff that is 10 times the patient's age in years for patients more than 50 years of age (age in years $\times$ 10 μg/L = cutoff). Incorporating age-adjusted D-dimer cutoffs into clinical practice is likely to become standard over the next few years.

The use of the Wells Score in older patients is less accurate than in younger patients, likely because of a change in case mix with an exclusively older population. In a study with nearly 300 patients more than 60 years of age, 44% living in a nursing home, the Wells Score had a failure rate of 6% at 3 months.[29]

In considering computed tomography (CT), the risks of radiation exposure in older patients is minimal and the risks of contrast-induced acute kidney injury is more substantial. In patients with acute or chronic kidney disease, using intravenous contrast can be avoided by pursuing a compression ultrasonography strategy. In patients with suspected PE, the presence of a proximal deep vein thrombosis has a positive likelihood ratio of 42 for PE, and the imaging work-up can be stopped at this point.[30] However, the converse is not true, and a negative compression ultrasonography does not mean that PE has been excluded. If the patient continues to have contraindications to CT imaging, V/Q studies should be considered. However, nondiagnostic V/Q studies are even more common in older patients than in younger patients. Patients with equivocal diagnostic evaluations require serial compression ultrasonography in 1 week.[30]

The management of PE in older patients is not very different from that in younger patients, although they are more likely to experience adverse effects of systemic anticoagulation.

ACUTE HEART FAILURE

Emergency departments are the first entry into the health care system for 80% of patients with acute HF. Emergency physicians negotiate many of the initial decisions regarding treatment options and risk stratification for acute HF.[35] HF accounts for 1 million annual emergency department visits in the United States.[36] Decompensated

HF can present in many ways. The easiest to recognize, acute pulmonary edema, accounts for between 25% and 40% of acute HF. Between 30% and 40% of patients with acute HF also have an acute coronary syndrome. Hypertensive acute HF accounts for about 25% of acute HF, and often presents with symptoms of pulmonary congestion.[35] In-hospital mortality from acute pulmonary edema is high (10%–20%), especially if acute pulmonary edema is associated with an acute myocardial infarction.[37] Other clinical features that are associated with increased in-hospital mortality from acute decompensated HF include anemia, systolic hypotension, and a reduced ejection fraction.[38] Other large registry studies have confirmed that advanced age and renal impairment are significant contributors to HF-increased mortality.[35] For all patients, the 12-month mortality is nearly 30% following an episode of acute pulmonary edema.[39]

The first challenge for the emergency physician is to establish that HF is the cause of acute dyspnea. However, the mimics of acute HF may also precipitate acute HF. Acute HF mimics include most of the causes of acute dyspnea, including pneumonia, COPD, and PE, and it can be difficult to establish which is the dominant disorder. Historical factors that support a diagnosis of HF include history of HF; orthopnea; paroxysmal nocturnal dyspnea; and medication or dietary noncompliance, especially of HF medications and salt intake. Physical findings that support a diagnosis of HF as a cause for acute dyspnea include increased venous pressures, particularly jugular venous distension and symmetric peripheral pitting edema. Pulmonary rales or crackles suggest the diagnosis of HF. In patients who have sufficient edema in the bronchioles, wheezing may be heard, which makes it difficult to distinguish pulmonary edema from a COPD exacerbation. Bedside ultrasonography can be used to look for evidence of interstitial edema and an assessment of cardiac contractility. Electrocardiogram (ECG) changes suggestive of acute ischemia, previous infarction, or ventricular hypertrophy add to the clinical suspicion but there is no diagnostic ECG criteria for acute HF. Increased troponin levels are suggestive, and an acutely increased natriuretic peptide level is strongly suggestive of acute HF.[35]

Treatment of HF is based initially on a symptom-based approach and then tailored therapy based on the precipitants or predisposing factors.[35] In general, the relief of symptoms in acute HF focuses on the relief of dyspnea.

Interventions that have proved useful in the symptomatic management of dyspnea associated with acute HF in the emergency department are positive pressure ventilation delivered via either continuous positive airway pressure (CPAP), bilevel positive pressure ventilation, or via endotracheal tube. In patients with acute pulmonary edema, NIV delivered by any method is associated with reduced symptoms and improved biochemical markers but NIV has no effect on short-term mortality compared with standard oxygen therapy.[37]

Standard therapy for acute dyspnea in HF includes oxygen, diuresis, and vasodilators. Intravenous diuretics are commonly used in the initial management for acute pulmonary edema, usually at or greater than the equivalent long-term oral dose, and titrated down to control symptoms.[36] Diuretics are particularly useful for patients with fluid overload, but most patients with acute pulmonary edema do not have fluid overload. Most patients with acute pulmonary edema have an acute increase in systemic vascular resistance and a vasodilator therapy is appropriate. Nitrate therapy, especially high-dose nitrate therapy, does have a proven benefit in acute HF.[35]

Excluding reversible precipitants of acute HF in the emergency department is important. This process commonly includes identifying acute coronary syndrome and arrhythmias, and uncommonly identifying acute valvular conditions.

NONINVASIVE VENTILATION

NIV consists of the delivery of ventilator support or positive pressure ventilation without endotracheal intubation, usually through a mask.[26] The most common modality for NIV is Continuous Positive Airway Pressure (CPAP) and Noninvasive Positive Pressure Ventilation (NPPV).

The more recent use of high-flow nasal cannula (HFNC) provides high flows of oxygen but does not offer formal pressure support. Although NIV is used in many settings, including in the postoperative period and after prolonged intubation, this article is limited to the role of NIV in the emergency department to manage acute respiratory failure. There is excellent evidence to support the use of NIV in acute respiratory failure in the emergency department. The two most common conditions for which NIV is commonly used are acute COPD exacerbations and acute pulmonary edema, both of which are much more commonly encountered in the older patient population.

In addition, there is emerging evidence for, and widespread use of, NIV as a short-term bridging technique in the 10 to 15 minutes before, and during endotracheal intubation in the emergency department in certain clinical situations.[40,41] In this situation, the expected course is that the patient still requires intubation, and NIV is used as a bridge to improved oxygenation, and to facilitate resuscitation before intubation.

CPAP provides continuous positive intrathoracic pressure but does not provide any inspiratory support.[26] CPAP is particularly useful in conditions characterized by acute hypoxic respiratory failure. CPAP has been used since the mid 1980s to manage acute pulmonary edema.

NPPV includes all of the modalities of NIV, including those with a set respiratory rate. NPPV provides inspiratory support and is particularly useful in conditions with acute hypercapnic respiratory failure. NPPV is often referred to by the commercial name of BiPAP (bilevel positive airway pressure).

HFNC, although not specifically providing inspiratory support, may be of value in older patients. HFNC is not NIV as traditionally described, because there is no true positive pressure. Technically, it is providing increased flow with variable pressure. There are 3 postulated mechanisms of action of HFNC: washout of pharyngeal dead space, reduction of upper airway resistance, and provision of a low level of intrathoracic pressure.[26] HFNC is easy to tolerate, and offers patients the ability to speak with family and loved ones.

NIV has been proved to be useful in acute respiratory failure[25–28] and should be used early in the patient's emergency department course. There is good evidence to suggest that early application of NIV is associated with fewer treatment failures resulting in endotracheal intubation. NIV is particularly helpful in COPD exacerbations and acute pulmonary edema.

The contraindications to the use of NIV are relative and absolute. Absolute contraindications include respiratory arrest, upper airway obstruction, inability to protect the airway with loss of airway (bulbar) reflexes, copious oral secretions, sputum, hemorrhage or emesis, and patient refusal. When considering NIV as a short-term bridging technique, absence of airway protection is a relative contraindication, because the medical team does not leave the patient's bedside. Relative contraindications to NIV include hemodynamic instability, patient agitation and inability to tolerate the mask, partial loss of airway reflexes, swallowing impairment, excessive secretions, multisystem organ failure (one other system in addition to respiratory failure), and rapidly progressive respiratory failure (including adult respiratory distress syndrome).[26]

In older patients, the use of NIV becomes particularly attractive in acute respiratory failure. NIV has the advantage in critically ill older patients of offering full respiratory support without the disadvantages of endotracheal intubation. In the emergency department, the use of NIV can facilitate discussions of goals of care with patients and their families. Unlike patients with endotracheal intubation, patients who are receiving NIV are able to take intermittent breaks from the ventilator, and can speak with family members and even take small amounts of oral nourishment. Note that older patients with do-not-intubate orders often do well on NIV, and studies have shown survival of 50% to 75% from the acute episode.[26,42] NIV is compatible with palliative care goals for relief of acute or severe dyspnea. NIV can be used in patients who are already receiving hospice care, or are being considered for hospice therapy, because health care providers or family members can speak directly with the patient at the same time that acute relief of symptoms is being provided. Patients on hospice may come to the emergency department with acute dyspnea, and NIV remains appropriate for these patients for relief of their symptoms.[43]

SUMMARY

Acute dyspnea in older patients is a common presentation to the emergency department. Acute dyspnea in older adults is often the consequence of multiple overlapping disorders, such as pneumonia precipitating acute HF. Emergency physicians must be comfortable managing patients with acute dyspnea of uncertain cause and varying goals of care. In addition to the important role NIV plays as full resuscitation, NIV can be useful as method of providing supportive care while more information is gathered from the patient and the patient's loved ones.

REFERENCES

1. Colby SO, Ortman JM. Projections of the size and composition of the U.S. population: 2014 to 2060. Population estimates and projections. Washington, DC: U.S. Census Bureau 2014.
2. United NationsDepartment of Economic and Social Affairs, Population Division. World population prospects: the 2010 revision, volume I: comprehensive tables. 2011. ST/ESA/SER.A/313.
3. Thannickal VJ, Murthy M, Balch WE, et al. Blue journal conference. Aging and susceptibility to lung disease. Am J Respir Crit Care Med 2015;191(3):261–9.
4. Gooneratne NS, Patel NP, Corcoran A. Chronic obstructive pulmonary disease diagnosis and management in older adults. J Am Geriatr Soc 2010;58(6): 1153–62.
5. Banerjee S. Multimorbidity—older adults need health care that can count past one. Lancet 2015;385(9968):587–9.
6. Lowery EM, Brubaker AL, Kuhlmann E, et al. The aging lung. Clin Interv Aging 2013;8:1489–96.
7. Wang YC, McPherson K, Marsh T, et al. Health and economic burden of the projected obesity trends in the USA and the UK. Lancet 2011;378(9793):815–25.
8. Dixon AE, Lundblad LK, Suratt BT. The weight of obesity on lung health. Pulm Pharmacol Ther 2013;26(4):403–4.
9. Sideleva O, Black K, Dixon AE. Effects of obesity and weight loss on airway physiology and inflammation in asthma. Pulm Pharmacol Ther 2013;26(4):455–8.
10. Sideleva O, Suratt BT, Black KE, et al. Obesity and asthma: an inflammatory disease of adipose tissue not the airway. Am J Respir Crit Care Med 2012;186(7): 598–605.
11. Pop-Vicas A, Gravenstein S. Influenza in the elderly: a mini-review. Gerontology 2011;57(5):397–404.

12. D'Mello T, Brammer L, Blanton L, et al. Update: influenza activity–United States, September 28, 2014-February 21, 2015. MMWR Morb Mortal Wkly Rep 2015; 64(8):206–12.

13. Thompson WW, Shay DK, Weintraub E, et al. Influenza-associated hospitalizations in the United States. JAMA 2004;292(11):1333–40.

14. Antiviral drugs for seasonal influenza 2014-2015. JAMA 2015;313(4):413–4.

15. Osterholm MT, Kelley NS, Sommer A, et al. Efficacy and effectiveness of influenza vaccines: a systematic review and meta-analysis. Lancet Infect Dis 2012;12(1): 36–44.

16. Tiruvoipati R, Ong K, Gangopadhyay H, et al. Hypothermia predicts mortality in critically ill elderly patients with sepsis. BMC Geriatr 2010;10:70.

17. Lim WS, van der Eerden MM, Laing R, et al. Defining community acquired pneumonia severity on presentation to hospital: an international derivation and validation study. Thorax 2003;58(5):377–82.

18. Towards better management of COPD. Lancet 2015;385(9979):1697.

19. Albertson TE, Louie S, Chan AL. The diagnosis and treatment of elderly patients with acute exacerbation of chronic obstructive pulmonary disease and chronic bronchitis. J Am Geriatr Soc 2010;58(3):570–9.

20. Global Strategy for the Diagnosis, Management and prevention of COPD, Global Initiative for Chronic Obstructive Lung Disease (GOLD). 2015. Available at: http://www.goldcopd.org/guidelines-global-strategy-for-diagnosis-management.html. Accessed May 11, 2015.

21. Decramer M, Janssens W, Miravitlles M. Chronic obstructive pulmonary disease. Lancet 2012;379(9823):1341–51.

22. COPD: improving prevention and care. Lancet 2015;385(9971):830.

23. Woodruff PG, Agusti A, Roche N, et al. Current concepts in targeting chronic obstructive pulmonary disease pharmacotherapy: making progress towards personalised management. Lancet 2015;385(9979):1789–98.

24. El Moussaoui R, Roede BM, Speelman P, et al. Short-course antibiotic treatment in acute exacerbations of chronic bronchitis and COPD: a meta-analysis of double-blind studies. Thorax 2008;63(5):415–22.

25. Hess DR. Noninvasive ventilation for acute respiratory failure. Respir Care 2013; 58(6):950–72.

26. Mas A, Masip J. Noninvasive ventilation in acute respiratory failure. Int J Chron Obstruct Pulmon Dis 2014;9:837–52.

27. Cabrini L, Landoni G, Oriani A, et al. Noninvasive ventilation and survival in acute care settings: a comprehensive systematic review and metaanalysis of randomized controlled trials. Crit Care Med 2015;43(4):880–8.

28. Hess DR. The evidence is in: noninvasive ventilation saves lives. Crit Care Med 2015;43(4):927–9.

29. Schouten HJ, Geersing G-J, Oudega R, et al. Accuracy of the Wells Clinical Prediction Rule for Pulmonary Embolism in Older Ambulatory Adults. J Am Geriatr Soc 2014;62(11):2136–41.

30. Righini M, Le Gal G, Bounameaux H. Venous thromboembolism diagnosis: unresolved issues. Thromb Haemost 2014;113(3):1184–92.

31. Righini M, Van Es J, Den Exter PL, et al. Age-adjusted D-dimer cutoff levels to rule out pulmonary embolism: the ADJUST-PE study. JAMA 2014;311(11): 1117–24.

32. Polo Friz H, Pasciuti L, Meloni DF, et al. A higher D-dimer threshold safely rules-out pulmonary embolism in very elderly emergency department patients. Thromb Res 2014;133(3):380–3.

33. Kirschner J, Kline J. Annals of Emergency Medicine Journal Club. Is it time to raise the bar? Age-adjusted D-dimer cutoff levels for excluding pulmonary embolism: answers to the July 2014 Journal Club questions. Ann Emerg Med 2014; 64(6):678–83.

34. Jaconelli T, Crane S. BET 2: should we use an age adjusted D-dimer threshold in managing low risk patients with suspected pulmonary embolism? Emerg Med J 2015;32(4):335–7.

35. Christ M, Mueller C. Call to action: initiation of multidisciplinary care for acute heart failure begins in the Emergency Department. Eur Heart J Acute Cardiovasc Care 2015. [Epub ahead of print].

36. Collins S, Storrow AB, Albert NM, et al. Early management of patients with acute heart failure: state of the art and future directions. A consensus document from the Society for Academic Emergency Medicine/Heart Failure Society of America Acute Heart Failure Working Group. J Card Fail 2015;21(1):27–43.

37. Gray A, Goodacre S, Newby DE, et al. Noninvasive ventilation in acute cardiogenic pulmonary edema. N Engl J Med 2008;359(2):142–51.

38. Karasek J, Widimsky P, Ostadal P, et al. Acute heart failure registry from high-volume university hospital ED: comparing European and US data. Am J Emerg Med 2012;30(5):695–705.

39. Goodacre S, Gray A, Newby D, et al. Health utility and survival after hospital admission with acute cardiogenic pulmonary oedema. Emerg Med J 2011;28(6):477–82.

40. Weingart SD. Preoxygenation, reoxygenation, and delayed sequence intubation in the emergency department. J Emerg Med 2011;40(6):661–7.

41. Weingart SD, Levitan RM. Preoxygenation and prevention of desaturation during emergency airway management. Ann Emerg Med 2012;59(3):165–75.e1.

42. Vargas N, Vargas M, Galluccio V, et al. Non-invasive ventilation for very old patients with limitations to respiratory care in half-open geriatric ward: experience on a consecutive cohort of patients. Aging Clin Exp Res 2014;26(6):615–23.

43. Lowery DS, Quest TE. Emergency medicine and palliative care. Clin Geriatr Med 2015;31(2):295–303.

Noninvasive Ventilation for the Emergency Physician

Michael G. Allison, MD[a], Michael E. Winters, MD[b],*

KEYWORDS

- Noninvasive ventilation • Acute respiratory failure
- Continuous positive airway pressure • Bilevel positive airway pressure
- High flow nasal cannula

KEY POINTS

- Bilevel positive airway pressure (BPAP) should be used in all cases of moderate to severe respiratory failure owing to exacerbations of chronic obstructive pulmonary disease.
- Continuous positive airway pressure or BPAP can be used in patients with acute exacerbations of cardiogenic pulmonary edema.
- Noninvasive monitoring (NIV) can be attempted in patients with asthma, traumatic respiratory failure, respiratory failure associated with immunosuppression, and community-acquired pneumonia.
- High-flow nasal cannula is an emerging therapy that may be useful to treat hypoxic respiratory failure.
- Patients started on NIV should be monitored closely. Signs and symptoms should be evaluated after 1 hour of NIV to determine success or failure of therapy.

INTRODUCTION

Emergency physicians (EPs) routinely evaluate and manage patients with acute respiratory failure (ARF). Noninvasive ventilation (NIV) delivers positive pressure ventilation through a tight-fitting mask and is an invaluable tool in the treatment of select emergency department (ED) patients with ARF. The use of NIV is associated with decreased rates of intubation and mortality.[1,2] Importantly, the use of NIV requires knowledge of appropriate patient selection, modes of delivery, selection of the correct amount of positive pressure, and appropriate methods of monitoring the patient.

Disclosures: The authors have no financial disclosures to report.
[a] Critical Care Medicine, St. Agnes Hospital, 900 South Caton Avenue, Baltimore, MD 21229, USA; [b] Emergency Medicine/Internal Medicine/Critical Care Program, University of Maryland School of Medicine, 110 South Paca Street, 6th Floor, Suite 200, Baltimore, MD 21201, USA
* Corresponding author.
E-mail address: mwinters@umem.org

Inappropriate and indiscriminate use of NIV can be fraught with pitfalls in patient care. It is imperative that the EP be knowledgeable about the use of NIV in ED patients with ARF. This article discusses the primary modes of NIV, traditional and novel applications of NIV, and practical considerations when initiating NIV.

MODES OF NONINVASIVE VENTILATION

There are 2 modes of NIV: continuous positive airway pressure (CPAP) and bilevel positive airway pressure (BPAP). In CPAP, the provider sets a single pressure that is applied during all phases of the respiratory cycle; it is analogous to the positive end-expiratory pressure (PEEP) set during invasive mechanical ventilation, and often these terms are used interchangeably. CPAP is most useful for patients who primarily have hypoxic respiratory failure. In contrast with CPAP, BPAP delivers 2 levels of pressure to the patient: inspiratory positive airway pressure (IPAP) and expiratory positive airway pressure (EPAP). EPAP is analogous to the pressure that patients receive during CPAP; in BPAP modes, EPAP and PEEP are typically used interchangeably. When a breath is initiated in BPAP, the patient receives the set IPAP. The IPAP has 2 components: the EPAP and the pressure support (PS) that is provided in addition to the EPAP. The additive pressures of EPAP and PS equal the IPAP (**Table 1**). BPAP can be useful for patients with both hypercapnic and hypoxic respiratory failure.

Recently, the high-flow nasal cannula (HFNC) has emerged as a method to deliver NIV through a nasal cannula rather than a tight-fitting face mask. HFNC devices deliver humidified oxygen at high flow rates to achieve high oxygen concentrations. The device has been better studied in patients with hypoxic respiratory failure, but there remains interest in using it for hypercapnic respiratory failure. The manner in which HFNC affects pulmonary physiology, either through dead space washout, by applying some small level of positive airway pressure, or another unknown mechanism, remains incompletely understood.[3]

PHYSIOLOGIC CHANGES WITH NONINVASIVE VENTILATION

To provide comprehensive care to critically ill patients, it is important for the EP to understand the pulmonary and cardiovascular changes that occur with NIV. The goal of NIV is to decrease the patient's work of breathing and improve pulmonary gas exchange. Often, a gestalt visual assessment of respiratory effort is used to describe the work of breathing. However, it is actually determined by a complicated

Table 1
Common acronyms in noninvasive ventilation

Acronym	Definition
NIV	Noninvasive ventilation
CPAP	Continuous positive airway pressure
BPAP	Bilevel positive airway pressure
PEEP	Positive end-expiratory pressure
iPEEP	Intrinsic positive end-expiratory pressure
EPAP	End positive expiratory pressure (= PEEP)
PS	Pressure support
IPAP	Inspiratory positive airway pressure (= PS + PEEP or PS + EPAP)
HFNC	High-flow nasal cannula

physiologic calculation that involves tidal volume and airway pressure. When positive pressure is applied, the work of breathing can decrease by 60% through several different mechanisms.[4] Application of CPAP or PEEP reduces the work of breathing by counteracting the patient's intrinsic PEEP. PS reduces work of breathing by decreasing the patient's contribution to the transpulmonary pressure during inspiration. PS and PEEP help to overcome atelectasis, decrease oxygen consumption by the respiratory muscles, and improve expiratory tidal volumes.[4] These changes improve ventilation–perfusion matching (V/Q), improve oxygenation, and allow more effective carbon dioxide removal.

A positive pressure breath affects the circulatory system by altering the dynamics of intrathoracic pressure. Increases in intrathoracic pressure impede venous return and reliably decrease the effective preload. For patients who are preload dependent, this change from negative pressure to positive pressure breathing can result in hypotension. Increases in intrathoracic pressure also assist the left ventricle by lowering cardiac afterload. By providing positive intrathoracic pressure, the left ventricle has less transmural wall stress during systole, allowing the myocardium to work more efficiently. Circulatory changes occurring with the addition of positive pressure ventilation can decrease both preload and afterload; this can be helpful in cases of acute cardiogenic pulmonary edema (ACPE), but must be applied cautiously in patients who might be preload dependent.

TRADITIONAL APPLICATIONS OF NONINVASIVE VENTILATION
Chronic Obstructive Pulmonary Disease

Acute exacerbations of chronic obstructive pulmonary disease (COPD) traditionally carried a high mortality rate—up to 33% of patients admitted to the hospital died despite appropriate therapy.[5–9] Patients with COPD have an expiratory airflow limitation owing to the collapse of small and medium-sized airways. When patients have acute exacerbations of COPD, they have difficulty with gas exchange and therefore retain carbon dioxide. Historically, the treatment of acute exacerbations of COPD consisted of the administration of bronchodilators, systemic corticosteroids, supplemental oxygen, and antibiotics. When all measures failed, patients were intubated and mechanically ventilated. Mortality rates and the frequency of intubation for patients with hypercapnic respiratory failure decreased once NIV became an option for treatment.

For patients with acute exacerbations of COPD, NIV is one of the most effective treatments to improve patient outcome. The mortality benefit of NIV has been assessed in a number of randomized controlled trials. A Cochrane review evaluated 10 studies that looked at patient mortality when NIV was used for COPD exacerbations. There was a significant benefit, with a number needed to treat (NNT) of just 10 to improve the mortality rate.[1]

With the development of NIV, practitioners recognized that using this therapy before patients reach the extremes of respiratory distress obviated the need for endotracheal intubation in many cases. The same Cochrane review examined the role of NIV to prevent endotracheal intubation in respiratory failure from COPD and found an NNT of just 4.[1] One in 4 patients was spared the need for sedation and invasive mechanical ventilation, which decreases the likelihood of a variety of ventilator-associated conditions that increase patient morbidity. Other outcomes shown to improve with the early application of NIV for COPD exacerbations include decreased hospital duration of stay, decreased complications, and improvements in pH, respiratory rate, and partial pressure of carbon dioxide in arterial blood ($Paco_2$).[1] BPAP was the primary mode of NIV in the studies examined by this Cochrane review. No high-quality studies have evaluated CPAP for COPD. Recent guidelines on the use of NIV support the use of BPAP for patients with COPD and pH of less than 7.35.[10] NIV in the form of BPAP should be started early in the treatment of ED patients with acute COPD exacerbations.

Acute Cardiogenic Pulmonary Edema

Exacerbation of acute congestive heart failure resulting in ACPE is a leading cause of ARF in EDs in the United States. The in-hospital mortality rate for patients with ACPE can be as high as 12%.[11] A growing body of literature supports the use of NIV in patients with ACPE.

In patients with or without existing cardiomyopathy, increased left ventricular end-diastolic pressures cause the left atrium to pump against an increased load. As the atrium becomes overwhelmed, an increased hydrostatic pressure gradient is created within the pulmonary arterial and venous systems. Eventually, the pulmonary interstitium becomes overloaded, resulting in alveolar collapse and widening of the area reserved for diffusion of gases. Therapy for ACPE is aimed at reducing cardiac preload, reducing afterload, removing excess volume, and recruiting areas of lung with V/Q mismatch.

Initial studies on the use of NIV for ACPE were performed in the 1930s; however, subsequent investigations shifted focus to more invasive ventilatory strategies. It was not until the publication of several case series in the 1970s that interest in NIV for ACPE resurfaced.[12] Clinical practice guidelines now strongly recommend the use of NIV for ACPE.[10] Similar to patients with acute COPD exacerbations, patients presenting with ACPE have a lower mortality rate when NIV is initiated early in their management. A Cochrane systematic review and metaanalysis found an NNT of 13 to improve mortality when NIV was compared with standard therapy for ACPE.[2] Interestingly, when CPAP and BPAP were compared individually with standard therapy, only CPAP demonstrated a statistical improvement in mortality (with an NNT of 9). In contrast, when the metaanalysis compared CPAP with BPAP, no difference was found in the mortality rate.[2] Although the current literature is more robust for CPAP, EPs should feel comfortable initiating either CPAP or BPAP for patients with ACPE. It might be reasonable to choose a NIV modality based on the presence of hypercapnia. Patients with ACPE and hypercapnia both have better outcomes with BPAP, and patients with ACPE without hypercapnia will see the consistent benefits of CPAP.[2] The authors favor the use of BPAP in patients with ACPE and hypercapnia, whereas patients with ACPE without hypercapnia may derive benefit from CPAP.

In addition to mortality, NIV has been shown to improve other outcomes in patients with ACPE. A Cochrane review of 22 trials found a decreased rate of endotracheal intubation (NNT of 8), decreased the length of stay in the intensive care unit, and decreased respiratory rate among patients receiving NIV. Interestingly, there were no improvements in heart rate, systolic blood pressure, diastolic blood pressure, or mean arterial pressure.[2] There had been concern that BPAP, compared with CPAP, might increase the incidence of acute myocardial infarction in patients with ACPE, but recent reports do not support this association.

NOVEL APPLICATIONS OF NONINVASIVE VENTILATION
Asthma Exacerbations

Given the similarities between asthma and COPD with respect to obstructive airway pathophysiology, it seems logical that NIV would improve outcomes in patients with acute exacerbations of asthma. However, no studies have demonstrated improved morbidity or mortality rates from the use of NIV in patients with asthma.

Asthma is a disease marked by the pathologic triad of airflow obstruction, mucus hypersecretion, and bronchoconstriction. Exacerbations of asthma can be caused by infection, medication nonadherence, environmental allergens, and exposure to cigarette smoke. Treatment of the patient with an acute asthma exacerbation centers on the administration of inhaled bronchodilators and systemic corticosteroids. Additional therapies that can be considered include intramuscular bronchodilators, magnesium sulfate, helium–oxygen admixture, and NIV.

There is a dearth of literature on the use of NIV in acute asthma exacerbations. A 2012 Cochrane review on NIV for acute asthma exacerbations states that "this course of treatment remains controversial."[13] A 2011 clinical practice guideline from the Canadian Critical Care Trials Group "make(s) no recommendation about the use of noninvasive positive-pressure ventilation in patients who have an exacerbation of asthma, because of insufficient evidence."[10] No randomized trial has evaluated the use of CPAP in asthma patients. Three small, randomized trials evaluated BPAP in asthma. Holley and colleagues[14] compared 19 patients placed on BPAP for asthma with 16 patients who received standard therapy. None of the patients in this study died; 1 patient in the BPAP group and 2 in the control group required intubation. The study was stopped early owing to poor enrollment. In the second study, Soroksky and colleagues[15] compared BPAP with standard therapy in 15 patients. No patients died or were intubated. In the third study, Soma and colleagues[16] analyzed 26 patients who received BPAP compared with 14 patients in a control arm. No patients died or were intubated.

Although the benefit of NIV in asthma has not been demonstrated in large, multi-center randomized trials, no demonstrable harm from this intervention has been detected. Its routine use cannot be recommended, but, in select cases of severe asthma, NIV should be considered.

Traumatic Respiratory Failure

Patients with blunt chest injury are at high risk for respiratory failure. In the trauma patient, endotracheal intubation and mechanical ventilation are associated with high rates of ventilator-associated pneumonia and prolonged use of mechanical ventilation.[17] Observational trials and several small, randomized studies have assessed the use of NIV in blunt chest trauma, yielding mixed results. A 2013 systematic review concluded that the early use of NIV in blunt chest trauma could be considered.[18] This recommendation is based on 1 medium-sized randomized trial that had improved rates of intubation in patients with chest trauma and hypoxemia (ratio of arterial oxygen partial pressure to fractional inspired oxygen [P/F ratio] <200) when managed with NIV compared with a nonrebreather mask.[19] Patients who develop respiratory failure later in their course (after 48 hours) are unlikely to benefit from NIV, so its use is not recommended.[18] Select patients with thoracic trauma who have hypoxic respiratory failure within the first 48 hours after trauma might benefit from BPAP. The available evidence does not support NIV as rescue therapy in patients with chest trauma who develop respiratory failure.

Community-Acquired Pneumonia

There is great interest in using NIV for patients with community-acquired pneumonia (CAP) to avoid the complications of invasive mechanical ventilation. Unfortunately, the literature on NIV for patients with CAP has produced mixed results. Prospective trials have demonstrated failure rates as high as 50%.[20–26] Studies that demonstrated lower rates of intubation with NIV in CAP primarily included patients who had less severe disease and responded to initial medical therapy.[26] A single, randomized, controlled trial evaluating standard therapy and standard therapy plus NIV in 56 patients with CAP found no improvement in the mortality rate. Patients who received NIV did have lower rates of intubation and shorter lengths of stay in an intermediate care unit.[27] An additional randomized, controlled trial evaluated patients with ARF of varying causes. In this study, patients with CAP who were treated with NIV had lower intubation rates and a lower mortality rate in the intensive care unit.[28]

Results from additional studies have demonstrated less favorable results, causing confusion about the role of NIV in patients with respiratory failure from CAP. As a result of the ambiguity in evidence, current guidelines do not provide a recommendation about the use of NIV in CAP.[10] If it is used, patients with less severe disease who show an early response to therapy might achieve benefit from NIV. It should be used with caution in patients with CAP.

Immunocompromised Patients

Treatment of ARF in the immunocompromised patient is fraught with difficulty. Immunosuppressed patients are at high risk for infectious complications of endotracheal intubation and mechanical ventilation. In a cohort of solid organ transplant patients with respiratory failure, Antonelli and colleagues[29] demonstrated decreased rates of intubation and mortality in the intensive care unit in patients randomized to NIV compared with standard therapy. Hilbert and colleagues[30] compared NIV with standard therapy in immunocompromised patients with pneumonia. Patients who received NIV for 3 hours, followed by a 3-hour period without NIV, had fewer intubations and decreased mortality. More recent data from a multicenter database of patients with hematologic malignancies demonstrated similar mortality rates between patients treated initially with NIV and those treated initially with mechanical ventilation.[31] Importantly, more than 50% of patients treated initially with NIV did not require intubation. Based on the available evidence, NIV guidelines recommend the use of BPAP in immunosuppressed patients with pneumonia.[10] It is important to recognize that the rate of NIV failure is higher for this patient population compared with other diseases, such as exacerbations of COPD and ACPE.

Delayed Sequence Intubation

Endotracheal intubation of the critically ill patient with hypoxia is difficult and fraught with the potential for morbidity and mortality. Some practitioners use NIV after sedation to recruit areas of lung with shunt physiology to improve the chance of successful endotracheal intubation without further hypoxia.[32] A prospective case series in the ED setting describes the successful application of this technique in patients presenting with acute hypoxic respiratory failure.[33] Misinterpretation of this technique has led some to view it as a way to avoid intubation. It should be emphasized that this approach to the patient in respiratory failure is not meant as a way to avoid intubation, but as a mechanism to provide safer conditions for it. If the patient fails to improve or worsens, the clinician should be ready to perform immediate intubation; if the patient improves, a more controlled intubation can be attempted.

CONTROVERSIAL USES OF NONINVASIVE VENTILATION
Altered Mental Status

Altered mental status is often mentioned as an absolute or relative contraindication to NIV. An international consensus conference even recommended that NIV not be used in patients with a Glasgow Coma Scale score of less than 10.[34] The principle behind this dogma is that altered patients could be unable to protect their airway and thus are at risk for aspiration. Many of the larger studies on NIV have excluded patients with any evidence of altered mental status. However, 2 studies evaluated NIV in patients with varying levels of mentation. The first examined 958 patients who received NIV. Investigators retrospectively determined patients' Glasgow Coma Scale score at the time NIV was initiated. They then compared patients with a Glasgow Coma Scale score of less than 8 with those with a score of greater than 8. The rates of intubation and mortality did not differ between the 2 groups.[35] A second study of 80 patients evaluated only altered patients with COPD. In this study, there was no difference in outcome between altered patients with a low mental status and those with normal mental status.[36] Based on available evidence, it seems reasonable to attempt a trial of NIV in select patients with altered mentation. Importantly, the cause of the alteration in mental status might portend different outcomes when using NIV. In the limited literature that is available currently, the highest success rates of NIV were achieved in altered patients with an acute COPD exacerbation.

Acute Respiratory Distress Syndrome

The acute respiratory distress syndrome (ARDS) describes a constellation of findings in patients with ARF. The Berlin Definition of ARDS defines the syndrome as ARF that occurs over 7 days and is marked by the presence of bilateral opacities on radiographic imaging, a partial pressure of oxygen in arterial blood (Pao_2)/fraction of inspired oxygen (Fio_2) ratio of less than 300, the absence of left heart failure as a significant contributor to the respiratory failure, and the need for 5 cm H_2O of PEEP.[37] Patients with ARDS have a high mortality rate. Studies evaluating the use of NIV in patients with ARDS have shown failure rates of approximately 50%. ARDS is not diagnosed commonly in the ED, primarily because the constellation of clinical, laboratory, and radiographic findings is not apparent in the first hours of presentation. For the EP, NIV should not be used in the hypoxic patient who has a clinical picture consistent with ARDS.

PRACTICAL CONSIDERATIONS FOR INITIATING NONINVASIVE VENTILATION

Once a patient is selected for treatment with NIV, the EP must choose the mode of ventilation, the type of interface, the PEEP or CPAP level, the IPAP or PS level, and the Fio_2 (**Box 1**). The selection of the NIV mode primarily depends on the clinical indication. BPAP remains a viable option for all disease states, and CPAP remains a highly effective therapy for patients with ACPE.

The NIV interface is usually determined by the availability of masks. Five types are available: nasal masks, nasal pillows, full face masks, total face mask, and helmets. The 2 most common interfaces are nasal masks and full face masks.[38] Despite head-to-head comparisons, a comment from an article published more than 2 decades ago remains timely: "The optimal interface and ventilator design have not been determined, and these may differ among patients."[39] Patients often complain about the tightness of the interface when it is first applied. Caution should be used when providing any patient on NIV a sedative or hypnotic medication to improve compliance with therapy. Allowing the anxious patient to hold the mask in place while low amounts of PEEP are first applied (3–5 cm H_2O) is a technique these authors have used with some anecdotal success.

When setting CPAP or PEEP, a common practice is to begin with 5 cm H_2O. PEEP can be titrated every 10 to 15 minutes by increasing pressure by 2 cm H_2O, with a goal of improving the SpO_2 or Pao_2. It is reasonable to start higher, around 8 to 12 cm H_2O,

---

Box 1
Practical considerations when initiating NIV

1. Choose CPAP or BPAP modality based on indication

2. Select interface/mask depending on local availability

CPAP

3. Set CPAP 5–10 cm H_2O

4. Set Fio_2 between 0.4 and 1.0

5. Titrate pressure 2 cm H_2O every 5 min to effect

6. Titrate Fio_2 according to SaO_2 or ABG

BPAP

3. Set EPAP or PEEP 5–8 cm H_2O

4. Set PS (7–10 cm H_2O) or IPAP (12–15 cm H_2O)

5. Set Fio_2 between 0.4 and 1.0

5. Titrate pressures 2 cm H_2O every 5 min to effect

6. Titrate Fio_2 according to SaO_2 or ABG

Abbreviations: ABG, arterial blood gases; BPAP, bilevel positive airway pressure; CPAP, continuous positive airway pressure; EPAP, expiratory positive airway pressure; Fio_2, fraction of inspired oxygen; IPAP, inspiratory positive airway pressure; NIV, noninvasive ventilation; PEEP, positive end-expiratory pressure; PS, pressure support; SaO_2, oxygen saturation.

---

when providing CPAP therapy for ACPE (studies that found a benefit to CPAP used these initial levels).[2] Health care providers should be mindful of the influence of PEEP on cardiac preload, because rapid titration could result in hypotension. Inspiratory pressures are set using the IPAP or PS. Many of the higher quality studies in the aforementioned Cochrane reviews used IPAP settings of 12 to 15 cm H_2O, which equates to a PS of 7 to 10 above the set PEEP.[1,2] As peak inspiratory pressures approach 20 to 25 cm H_2O, the practitioner should be aware of the increasing chance for gastric insufflation. The lower esophageal sphincter tone in normal patients is about 25 cm H_2O and can be lower in critically ill patients. At these inspiratory pressure levels, the risks of inducing vomiting and subsequent aspiration should be weighed against further benefits of added PS or PEEP.

Fio_2 can be set anywhere in the range of 21% to 100%. For patients requiring an Fio_2 of greater than 80% while receiving a PEEP of 5 cm H_2O, it is reasonable to increase PEEP to 8 to 10 cm H_2O to recruit areas with physiologic shunting and decrease the theoretic risks of oxygen toxicity.[40]

PREDICTING THE SUCCESS OR FAILURE OF NONINVASIVE VENTILATION

Despite the early application of NIV, some patients eventually require endotracheal intubation and mechanical ventilation. Depending on the clinical indication for NIV, the likelihood of failure varies dramatically. As discussed, 80% of patients with acute exacerbations of COPD can be managed successfully with NIV, whereas 50% of immunocompromised patients may require intubation. Thus, clinical indication remains as a robust predictor of success.[20] The ability to predict which patients will fail NIV and require intubation is critical. Frequent reassessment of patients on NIV is necessary, and the clinical variables listed in **Table 2**, which indicate the likelihood of success or failure, should be assessed after 30 to 60 minutes of treatment.[20,41]

HIGH-FLOW NASAL CANNULA

Providing supplemental oxygen using a nasal cannula has been standard therapy for hypoxic patients for decades. The amount of supplemental oxygen delivered with a traditional nasal cannula ranges from 25% to 35%.[42] Beginning in the early

Table 2	
Predictors of the failure or success of NIV after 1 hour	
Failure	**Success**
Sepsis as a cause of the respiratory failure	Improving pH
ARDS	Improving $Paco_2$
Higher severity score (SAPS II)	Improving Pao_2/Fio_2 ratio

Abbreviations: ARDS, acute respiratory distress syndrome; Fio_2, fraction of inspired oxygen; NIV, noninvasive ventilation; $Paco_2$, partial pressure of carbon dioxide in arterial blood; Pao_2, partial pressure of oxygen in arterial blood; SAPS, Simplified Acute Physiology Score.

1990s, there was interest in using higher flow rates to produce a greater oxygen concentration through HFNC devices, which consist of a specialized nasal cannula, an oxygen delivery device, and a humidification system. Studies have tested humidified HFNC delivery systems against nonrebreather masks, finding that the HFNC system can deliver higher Fio_2 concentrations than nonrebreather masks at the same flow rates.[43] Commercial high-flow devices became available in the early 2000s and their use in adult patients has expanded dramatically since that time.

As use of HFNC devices became more common, questions were raised about the ability of this modality to provide a level of positive airway pressure. Initial reports evaluated healthy adult volunteers to quantify the capability of HFNC devices to generate positive airway pressure.[44,45] In these studies, a pressure transducer was fitted to a nasopharyngeal catheter, which sat in the posterior pharyngeal space as the supplemental oxygen was provided. Groves and Tobin[44] varied the HFNC flow between 10 and 60 L/min and measured pressures when the subject's mouth was closed and open. The posterior pharyngeal pressures rose linearly from 3.7, 7.2, and 8.7 cm H_2O when respective flows of 20, 40, and 60 L/min were used. Pressure measurements obtained in a mouth open situation decreased to 1.4, 2.2, and 2.7 cm H_2O using the same levels of flow. The Park group maintained a constant 35 L/min flow and found the mean pharyngeal pressure to be 2.7 cm H_2O with the mouth closed and 1.2 cm H_2O when the mouth was open. In contrast with CPAP, the pressure waveform decreased to zero during inspiration.[45] These physiologic studies suggest that any positive pressure effect of HFNC is meager and dissipates with open mouth breathing and during inspiration.

HFNC systems have been used in a number of scenarios, and their effects on clinical variables have been reported in the literature based on observational studies and prospective comparisons with face mask devices. When used in patients with mild to moderate hypoxemia, HFNC devices are well-tolerated, provide a reliable improvement in Pao_2, and reduce patients' respiratory rate.[3] Oxygenation via an HFNC seems to be an attractive and viable option for patients with hypoxemic respiratory failure and in patients after cardiac surgery.[46,47] At present, these devices should not be used as first-line therapy for diseases such as COPD and ACPE, which clearly benefit from traditional NIV modalities; they are also an attractive option for patients with hypoxemic respiratory failure. Future studies will likely elucidate the indications for use of these systems.

SUMMARY

ARF is commonly encountered in the ED. Select patients with ARF can be managed effectively with NIV. The best evidence for use of NIV comes from patients presenting with acute exacerbations of COPD and ACPE. Less robust evidence is available for diseases such as asthma and immunocompromised respiratory failure; in these cases, a trial of NIV can be considered. Patients with diseases such as traumatic respiratory failure, ARDS, and CAP are not likely to benefit from NIV. BPAP and CPAP are the most commonly used modes of NIV, and practitioners should be aware of the beneficial and detrimental physiologic changes associated with their use. Oxygenation via HFNC is an attractive option to treat the hypoxic patient, but is not a replacement for NIV. Clinicians should be aware that failure of NIV is common, and its use requires vigilance and constant reassessment of the patient with respiratory failure.

REFERENCES

1. Ram FS, Picot J, Lightowler J, et al. Non-invasive positive pressure ventilation for treatment of respiratory failure due to exacerbations of chronic obstructive pulmonary disease. Cochrane Database Syst Rev 2004;(3):CD004104.
2. Vital FM, Saconato H, Laderia MT, et al. Non-invasive positive pressure ventilation (CPAP or bilevel NPPV) for cardiogenic pulmonary edema [review]. Cochrane Database Syst Rev 2013;(5):CD005351.
3. Ward JJ. High-flow oxygen administration by nasal cannula for adult and perinatal patients. Respir Care 2013;58:98–122.
4. Kallet RH, Diaz JV. The physiologic effects of noninvasive ventilation. Respir Care 2009;54:102–15.
5. Ambrosino N, Foglio K, Rubini F, et al. Non-invasive mechanical ventilation in acute respiratory failure due to chronic obstructive pulmonary disease: correlates for success. Thorax 1995;50:755–7.
6. Bott J, Carroll MP, Conway JH, et al. Randomised controlled trial of nasal ventilation in acute ventilatory failure due to chronic obstructive airways disease. Lancet 1993;341(8860):1555–7.
7. Brochard L, Mancebo J, Wysocki M, et al. Noninvasive ventilation for acute exacerbations of chronic obstructive pulmonary disease. N Engl J Med 1995;333:817–22.
8. Foglio C, Vitacca M, Quadri A, et al. Acute exacerbations in severe COLD patients. treatment using positive pressure ventilation by nasal mask. Chest 1992;101:1533–8.
9. Jeffery AA, Warren PM, Flenley DC. Acute hypercapnic respiratory failure in patients with chronic obstructive lung disease; risk factors and use of guidelines for management. Thorax 1992;47:34–40.
10. Keenan SP, Sinuff T, Burns KEA, et al. Clinical practice guidelines for the use of noninvasive positive-pressure ventilation and noninvasive continuous positive airway pressure in the acute care setting. CMAJ 2011;183:E195–214.
11. Roguin A, Behar D, Ben Ami H, et al. Long-term prognosis of acute pulmonary oedema—an ominous outcome. Eur J Heart Fail 2000;2:137–44.
12. Greenbaum D, Millen J, Eross B, et al. Continuous positive airway pressure without tracheal intubation in spontaneously breathing patients. Chest 1976;69:615–20.
13. Lim WJ, Mohammed Akram R, Carson KV, et al. Non-invasive positive pressure ventilation for treatment of respiratory failure due to severe acute exacerbations of asthma. Cochrane Database Syst Rev 2012;(12):CD004360.
14. Holley MT, Morrissey TK, Seaberg DC, et al. Ethical dilemmas in a randomized trial of asthma treatment: can Bayesian statistical analysis explain the results? Acad Emerg Med 2001;8:1128–35.

15. Soroksky A, Stav D, Shpirer I. A pilot, prospective, randomized, placebo-controlled trial of bilevel positive airway pressure in acute asthmatic attack. Chest 2003;123:1018–25.
16. Soma T, Hino M, Kida K, et al. A prospective and randomized study for improvement of acute asthma by non-invasive positive pressure ventilation (NPPV). Intern Med 2008;47:493–501.
17. Tyburski JG, Collinge JD, Wilson RF, et al. Pulmonary contusions: quantifying the lesions on chest x-ray films and the factors affecting prognosis. J Trauma 1999; 17:833–8.
18. Duggal A, Perez P, Golan E, et al. Safety and efficacy of noninvasive ventilation in patients with blunt chest trauma: a systematic review. Crit Care 2013;17:R142.
19. Hernandez G, Fernandez R, Lopez-Reina P, et al. Noninvasive ventilation reduces intubation in chest trauma-related hypoxemia: a randomized clinical trial. Chest 2010;137:74–80.
20. Antonelli M, Conti G, Moro ML, et al. Predictors of failure of noninvasive positive pressure ventilation in patients with acute hypoxemic respiratory failure: a multi-center study. Intensive Care Med 2001;27:1718–28.
21. Rana S, Jenad H, Gay PC, et al. Failure of noninvasive ventilation in patients with acute lung injury: observational cohort study. Crit Care 2006;10:R79.
22. Honrubia T, Garcia Lopez FJ, Franco N, et al. Noninvasive vs conventional mechanical ventilation in acute respiratory failure: a multicenter, randomized controlled trial. Chest 2005;128:3916–24.
23. Antro C, Merico F, Urbino R, et al. Noninvasive ventilation as a first-line treatment for acute respiratory failure: 'real-life' experience in the emergency department. Emerg Med J 2005;22:772–7.
24. Carron M, Freo U, Zorzi M, et al. Predictors of failure of noninvasive ventilation in patients with severe community-acquired pneumonia. J Crit Care 2010;25:540.e9–14.
25. Carrillo A, Gonzalez-Diaz G, Ferrer M, et al. Noninvasive ventilation in community-acquired pneumonia and severe acute respiratory failure. Intensive Care Med 2012;38:458–66.
26. Nicolini A, Ferraioli G, Ferrari-Bravo M, et al. Early noninvasive ventilation in community-acquired pneumonia. Clin Respir J 2014. [Epub ahead of print].
27. Confalonieri M, Potena A, Carbone G, et al. Acute respiratory failure in patients with severe community-acquired pneumonia: a prospective randomized evaluation of noninvasive ventilation. Am J Respir Crit Care Med 1999;160: 1585–9.
28. Ferrer M, Esquinas A, Leon M, et al. Noninvasive ventilation in severe hypoxemic respiratory failure: a randomized clinical trial. Am J Respir Crit Care Med 2003; 168:1438–44.
29. Antonelli M, Conti G, Bufi M, et al. Noninvasive ventilation for treatment of acute respiratory failure in patients undergoing solid organ transplantation. JAMA 2000; 283:235–41.
30. Hilbert G, Gruson D, Vargas F, et al. Noninvasive ventilation in immunosuppressed patients with pulmonary infiltrates, fever, and acute respiratory failure. N Engl J Med 2001;344:481–7.
31. Gristina GR, Antonelli M, Conti G, et al. Noninvasive versus invasive ventilation for acute respiratory failure in patients with hematologic malignancies: a 5-year multicenter observational survey. Crit Care Med 2011;39:2232–9.
32. Baillard C, Fosse JP, Sebbane M, et al. Noninvasive ventilation improves preoxygenation before intubation of hypoxic patients. Am J Respir Crit Care Med 2006; 174:171–7.

33. Weingart SD, Trueger NS, Wong N, et al. Delayed sequence intubation: a prospective observational study. Ann Emerg Med 2014;65:349–55.
34. Evans TW. International Consensus Conferences in Intensive Care Medicine: noninvasive positive pressure ventilation in acute respiratory failure. Organised jointly by the American Thoracic Society, the European Respiratory Society, the European Society of Intensive Care Medicine, and the Société de Réanimation de Langue Française, and approved by the ATS Board of Directors, December 2000. Intensive Care Med 2001;27:166–78.
35. Diaz GG, Alcaraz AC, Talavera JCP, et al. Noninvasive positive-pressure ventilation to treat hypercapnic coma secondary to respiratory failure. Chest 2005;127:952–60.
36. Scala R, Naldi N, Archinucci I, et al. Noninvasive positive pressure ventilation in patients with acute exacerbations of COPD and varying levels of consciousness. Chest 2005;128:1657–66.
37. The ARDS Definition Task Force. Acute respiratory distress syndrome: the Berlin definition. JAMA 2012;307:2526–33.
38. Antonelli M, Pennisi MA, Conti G. New advances in the use of noninvasive ventilation for acute hypoxaemic respiratory failure. Eur Respir J Suppl 2003;42:65s–71s.
39. Meyer TJ, Hill NS. Noninvasive positive pressure ventilation to treat respiratory failure. Ann Intern Med 1994;120:760–70.
40. Brower RG, Lanken PN, MacIntyre N, et al, Acute National Heart Lung and Blood Institute ARDS Clinical Trials Network. Higher versus lower positive end-expiratory pressures in patients with the acute respiratory distress syndrome. N Engl J Med 2004;351:327–36.
41. Anton A, Guell R, Gomez J, et al. Predicting the result of noninvasive ventilation in severe acute exacerbations of patients with chronic airflow limitation. Chest 2000;117:828–33.
42. Markovitz GH, Colthurst J, Storer TW, et al. Effective inspired oxygen concentration measured via transtracheal and oral gas analysis. Respir Care 2010;55:453–9.
43. Tiep BL, Barnett J, Schiffman G, et al. Maintaining oxygenation via demand oxygen delivery during rest and exercise. Respir Care 2002;47:887–92.
44. Groves N, Tobin A. High flow nasal oxygen generates positive airway pressure in adult volunteers. Aust Crit Care 2007;20:126–31.
45. Parke R, McGuinness S, Eccleston M. Nasal high flow oxygen delivers low level positive airway pressure. Br J Anaesth 2009;103:886–90.
46. Frat JP, Thille AW, Mercat A, et al. High-flow oxygen through nasal cannula in acute hypoxemic respiratory failure. N Engl J Med 2015;372(23):2185–96.
47. Stéphan F, Barrucand B, Petit P, et al. High-flow nasal oxygen vs noninvasive positive airway pressure in hypoxemic patients after cardiothoracic surgery: a randomized clinical trial. JAMA 2015;313(23):2331–9.

Emergency Department Treatment of the Mechanically Ventilated Patient

Rory Spiegel, MD[a], Haney Mallemat, MD[b],*

KEYWORDS

- Mechanical ventilation • Volume control • Pressure control
- Synchronized intermittent mandatory ventilation • Airway pressure release ventilation
- Pressure support ventilation

KEY POINTS

- Mechanical ventilation is a commonly used but sometimes poorly understood modality in the emergency department.
- In the modern emergency department, where patients remain under the care of the emergency physician for a longer duration, physicians must become comfortable with treating ventilated patients for extended periods.
- Emergency physicians need to understand how to initiate, titrate, and manage mechanical ventilation.
- Emergency physicians must have the ability to adapt ventilatory strategies for specific patients, understand the potential harms of mechanical ventilation, and take action to reduce their incidence.

HISTORY OF MECHANICAL VENTILATION

Mechanical ventilation has a long, storied history. Descriptions of positive-pressure ventilation can be found in the Old Testament, in writings dating from 800 BC. A passage from *Kings* 4:34 to 35 describes the Prophet Elisha performing mouth-to-mouth ventilation on a dying child[1]:

And he went up, and lay upon the child, and put his mouth upon his mouth, and his eyes upon his eyes, and his hands upon his hands: and stretched himself upon the child; and the flesh of the child waxed warm.

Disclosures: None.
The article was copyedited by Linda J. Kesselring, MS, ELS, the technical editor/writer in the Department of Emergency Medicine at the University of Maryland School of Medicine.
[a] Department of Emergency Medicine, Stony Brook Medical Center, 101 Nicolls Rd, Stony Brook, NY 11790, USA; [b] University of Maryland School of Medicine, 110 South Paca Street, 6th Floor, Suite 200, Baltimore, MD 21201, USA
* Corresponding author.
E-mail address: haney.mallemat@gmail.com

Emerg Med Clin N Am 34 (2016) 63–75
http://dx.doi.org/10.1016/j.emc.2015.08.005

Hippocrates described the process of endotracheal intubation in his book *Treatise on Air*, published in 460 BC: "One should introduce a cannula into the trachea along the jaw bone so that air can be drawn into the lungs."[1]

Despite these early forays into positive-pressure ventilation, our application of mechanical ventilation took a dark turn in England in the 18th century. Doctors used bellows and a long tube inserted in the rectum to blow smoke into a drowned patient's gastrointestinal tract. Their intention was to stimulate the failing myocardium and dry the recently submerged body from the inside.[2] As medical knowledge advanced, this practice lost favor because of its obvious absurdity. Although some would say our understanding of mechanical ventilation has grown immensely since that era, others would argue that we have merely learned the appropriate orifice through which to ventilate!

This article reviews the common modes of mechanical ventilation that emergency physicians are likely to experience in their practice, discusses the strengths and weaknesses of the various approaches, and proposes a strategy of how best to initiate and maintain mechanical ventilation in the wide range of patients who are intubated in the emergency department.

INTRODUCTION TO VARIABLES

In 1493, Paracelsus, a Swiss German renaissance physician, inserted a tube connected to fire bellows into a patient's mouth to assist with ventilation. A person pumped the bellows, delivering breaths to the patient. The force, rate, and timing of each breath were left to the prerogative of whoever was squeezing the bellows.[3] In modern ventilators, we have outsourced these tasks to a mechanical circuit with adjustable settings.

Imagine that you have just intubated a patient and now must provide adequate ventilator support. Instead of a modern ventilator, you have a turn-of-the-century bellows device. You also have an assistant, who will pump the device in your absence. How would you instruct him to ventilate your patient?

Management of Ventilation

Trigger

When should your eager assistant pump the bellows? After all, you cannot stand next to the bedside, commanding him to pump the bellows each time you want to give your patient some air. If you instructed him to pump the bellows once every 6 seconds, then your patient would receive a fixed respiratory rate independent of his or her own respiratory efforts. On the other hand, if you instructed your assistant to pump the bellows only when the patient initiated a spontaneous breath, you would simply be augmenting your patient's own respiratory rate. The trigger is simply the stimulus that notifies your assistant or the modern-day ventilator when to deliver a breath.[4,5]

Limit

Now that you have instructed your assistant when to pump the bellows, how much air should he deliver? Should he deliver the maximum volume the bellows contains, or would it be prudent to tailor the amount of gas delivered to the size and requirements of the patient? Traditionally, the quantity of breath delivered is controlled in 2 ways: volume controlled and pressure controlled. Volume-controlled ventilation delivers a fixed volume of gas with each breath.[4] But, in some cases, control over the volume of breath delivered is not ideal (discussed in more detail later). In such scenarios, the assistant should be instructed to pump the bellows until a specific pressure is reached on the manometer attached to the bellows device. Once this threshold is reached, he should halt his delivery, independent of the volume of gas delivered. This is pressure-controlled ventilation.[4]

Cycle

Finally, how fast do you instruct your assistant to deliver each breath? For example, if you have instructed him to deliver 10 breaths each minute, then he will pump the bellows once every 6 seconds. How long should it take for him to deliver the breath? Remember that your assistant must allow time for the patient to passively exhale. In our natural spontaneous breathing pattern, we spend much more time in exhalation than in inhalation. Therefore, we commonly ask our assistants and ventilators to deliver a breath quickly, allowing adequate time for exhalation. The relationship between these intervals is the inhalation-to-exhalation ratio (I/E). The I/E is controlled by 2 factors: first, the amount of time spent in each breath cycle (number of breaths taken per minute) and, second, the speed at which the breath is delivered. If we instruct our assistant to deliver 10 breaths per minute, then he has 6 seconds to complete every breath cycle. If he delivers each breath over a 2-second period, he has 4 seconds to allow for passive expiration. This yields an I/E ratio of 2/4 or ½. If I asked him to deliver 20 breaths per minute, then each breath cycle would only be 3 seconds long. If he continued to deliver each breath over a 2-second interval, he would only have 1 second for passive exhalation before he had to give the next breath. This would create an I/E of 2/1. If you instructed him to deliver his breaths twice as fast, he would have 2 seconds for passive exhalation, changing the I/E ratio to 1/2. Thus, changing the speed of inhalation directly affects the I/E ratio.[4]

A reduction in expiratory time is normally of little consequence, but it becomes a problem for patients with asthma or chronic obstructive pulmonary disease (COPD), in whom bronchoconstriction prolongs the expiratory phase.[4] Too short of an expiratory time in these patients results in retention of tidal volumes within the lung from a previous breath. The retention of volume within the chest (also known as intrinsic or auto positive end-expiratory pressure [PEEP]) can lead to hemodynamic problems (increased intrathoracic pressure and compression of the great vessels) and pulmonary complications such as barotrauma. Please note that PEEP is defined as positive pressure that exists within the tracheobronchial tree and the lungs at the end of expiration; in this example it can lead to a pathologic condition; however, as will be discussed, PEEP can be used beneficially when ventilating patients.

Management of Oxygenation

Fraction of inspired oxygen

Imagine that your assistant can fill his bellows from 2 sources. One source is 100% oxygen, the other is room air (21% oxygen). Your assistant is able to draw from both sources, giving him whatever concentration of oxygen you request. This concentration is expressed as a ratio, fraction of inspired oxygen (F_{IO_2}).[4]

Positive end-expiratory pressure

The PEEP is the measured pressure at the end of expiration. In our example, it is measured on the bellows manometer as the patient exhales. PEEP has 2 components: intrinsic PEEP, generated by the patient's own physiology and extrinsic PEEP, which is added to the system for therapeutic purposes. These 2 pressures are additive. In our case, we can increase the extrinsic PEEP of our system by asking our assistant to tighten a release valve that controls the rate at which gas is released from our system. Likewise, modern ventilators allow you to set the amount of extrinsic PEEP that will be present throughout the respiratory cycle.[4]

MODES OF VENTILATION

Now that we have established the variables that constitute a ventilatory strategy, we turn to the modes of ventilation commonly used in emergency departments and intensive care units.

Volume-Controlled Ventilation

Imagine that you have placed an opaque screen between the patient and your assistant and asked him to deliver a selected number of breaths per minute, at a given volume, with a set inspiratory flow rate. In this mode of ventilation, your assistant is detached from the patient's intrinsic respiratory efforts and will uniformly deliver the requested number of breaths at the desired volume. If the patient attempts to take a spontaneous breath, it will go unnoticed by the blinded assistant. Likewise, if the patient has yet to finish the previous breath's exhalation, your assistant will automatically deliver the subsequent breath despite this incomplete expiratory effort. This lack of synchrony can cause significant distress to the patient and, in some cases, serious lung injury. For the aforementioned reasons, it is not a recommended mode of ventilation in the emergency department, unless the patient is fully anesthetized and paralyzed.[3]

Volume Assist–Control Ventilation

Now imagine you have removed the screen separating your assistant and the patient but again ask your assistant to deliver a set volume of gas from the bellows. This time, you ask him to pump the bellows in synchrony with the patient's intrinsic breaths. Every time the patient begins to inspire, your assistant delivers a predetermined volume of air. As a safety mechanism, because you cannot stand at the bedside watching, you set a baseline respiratory rate, below which your assistant will pump the bellows independent of the patient's intrinsic efforts.[3]

This mode of ventilation creates a more natural ventilatory cycle for the patient, allowing him to control when a breath is initiated and forcing in breaths only when the patient's intrinsic rate of breathing is insufficient for ventilation. Despite allowing for the patient's own initiation of each breath, the process of mechanical ventilation can be a distressing experience, as the rest of the components of the ventilatory cycle are out of the patient's control. For example, if the patient wishes to take larger volumes of air than you have instructed your assistant to allow, generating enough inspiratory force to inhale the remainder can prove difficult because the patient is working against the resistance of the entire circuit. Likewise, if the rate at which you have instructed your assistant to deliver each breath is slower than the patient's natural inspiratory inclination, then the work of breathing naturally increases as the patient inhales against resistance.[3]

Pressure Control Ventilation

Similar to volume control ventilation, pressure control places a screen between your assistant and the patient. Again, you instruct your assistant to deliver a selected number of breaths per minute. But instead of instructing him to give a set volume of gas, you now instruct him to pump the bellows until the monometer reaches a specific pressure threshold. Your assistant will continue to deliver this breath at this pressure for 1 second (cycle time). At this point, he will cease breath delivery independent of the volume of gas delivered.[3] You are able to adjust the volume of gas delivered by adjusting the pressure and cycle time. If you instruct your assistant to pump his bellows at a higher continual pressure then the volume of gas delivered will be higher. Concordantly, if you instruct him to provide the same constant pressure for a longer duration (cycle time), this too will increase the volume of gas delivered.

Pressure Assist–Control Ventilation

Once again, you have removed the screen separating your assistant from the patient, instructing him to pump the bellows until the monometer reaches a given pressure value. You ask him to pump the bellows in synchrony with the patient's intrinsic breaths. Every time the patient begins to inspire, your assistant will pump the bellows until the predetermined pressure level is reached. As a safety mechanism, because you cannot stand at the bedside watching, you set a baseline respiratory rate, below which your assistant will pump the bellows independent of the patient's intrinsic efforts.[3]

Volume and pressure both have advantages and disadvantages in the determination of the quantity of gas delivered. A volume-controlled mode of ventilation ensures that your patient receives an exact amount of air with each breath. This approach can work against you, as the predetermined volume delivered does not take into account the clinical scenario. For example, say you have instructed your assistant to deliver 400 mL of volume with each breath to an asthmatic who has been intubated for respiratory failure. The patient is still paralyzed from the long-acting paralytic you gave during the intubation process, so you tell your assistant to pump the bellows once every 5 seconds (ie, a respiratory rate of 12). While you are away seeing other patients, your assistant does exactly as instructed. What your assistant does not notice is that, because of the patient's obstructive physiology, he is exhaling only 300 mL of gas after each breath. As your assistant indiscriminately pumps 400 mL, the patient is trapping 100 mL of air with each breath. The manometer on the bellows is rising with each pump, and your assistant notices that it is becoming increasingly hard to deliver the allotted volume of air. But he is fastidious in his duties and continues to deliver 400 mL of air. This is the phenomenon of breath stacking, which is just as likely to occur with a volume control mode on a modern ventilator. This example highlights the major shortcoming of using volume goals exclusively to ventilate patients. In certain pathologic circumstances, a volume-guided approach to ventilation can be deleterious for the patient, as it does not account for physiologic states that cause high pressures during positive-pressure ventilation. In cases of obstructive physiology, continual delivery of a set volume of air without taking note of the expiratory volume can lead to breath stacking, pneumothorax, and even death. Additionally, in patients with acute lung injury, the intrinsic elasticity of the lung can be damaged, causing "stiff lung" and leading to acute respiratory distress syndrome (ARDS).[6] Ventilating patients at normal lung volumes can further damage their already-injured lung parenchyma. If you continue to ventilate these patients without accounting for the high alveolar pressures created by their pathology, you risk contributing to their disease iatrogenically.[3]

Now you are savvy to the harms of an unchecked volume-controlled method of ventilation in a patient with asthma. You instruct your assistant to pump the bellows until the monometer reaches 40 mm Hg and to continue delivering this pressured breath for 1 second, at which point he will stop. You walk away, satisfied that you have ensured the safety of your patient's lungs. But when you return a short time later, you find your patient is hypoxic and cyanotic despite your assistant doing just as you instructed. What happened this time? Our assistant had dutifully followed your instruction to the letter. He initiated a breath once every 5 seconds and delivered only enough air to reach a certain pressure limit on the manometer. Because your patient is showing significant obstructive pathology, the peak ventilator pressures will be elevated. Therefore, each time your assistant initiated a breath, the manometer quickly reached the predefined pressure limit, but little air was delivered to the patient. Not surprisingly, the patient's carbon dioxide (CO_2) level began to increase quickly, because no ventilation was being delivered. Eventually, even the patient's partial pressure of oxygen, arterial (Pao_2) level began to decrease. This example shows that a purely pressure-guided method of mechanical ventilation can be equally problematic.[3]

Pressure-Regulated Volume Control

Now that we have effectively mismanaged our patient in several ways, we must find a way to ensure that he receives adequate volumes of gas while minimizing harm to his lung parenchyma caused by increased alveolar pressures. You instruct your assistant to pump the bellows once every 5 seconds and deliver a breath using the manometer (pressure controlled). Additionally, you inform him of the desired volume you wish the patient to receive. To accomplish this, your assistant will deliver a test breath using a specific pressure and observe the volume of gas it delivers. If this volume is more than or less than the specified volume, your assistant will adjust the pressure used for the subsequent breath. He will continue to adjust his pressures to deliver the desired volume of gas.

This example describes the pressure-regulated volume control mode of ventilation, a pressure-controlled approach in which you assign the volume of gas delivered, the trigger to initiate ventilation, the PEEP, Fio_2 levels, and a peak pressure limit. A more appropriate name for this mode of ventilation would be pressure control, volume guaranteed ventilation. This method of ventilation allows you to control both the pressure and volume of gas during ventilation.[3]

Synchronized Intermittent Mandatory Ventilation

Some clinicians have suggested that even pressure-regulated volume control modes of ventilation create a ventilatory environment that is unnatural to the intubated patient. Although the patient guides the initiation of each breath, the inspiratory rate and volume are determined by the ventilator. If either of them is not congruent with the patient's needs, ventilator dysynchrony is produced. Synchronized intermittent mandatory ventilation can ameliorate these problems. Similar to the previously described modes, you assign a specific tidal volume, respiratory rate, inspiratory flow rate, Fio_2, and PEEP. The assistant is instructed to pump the bellows a given number of times per minute, delivering the amount of gas at the determined flow rate with each breath.[3] You then set the respiratory rate at a frequency below which the patient would typically breathe. You again place the screen between your assistant and the patient, this time providing an escape valve in the circuit that allows the patient to take independent breaths not determined by the bellows. Now the patient will receive 2 forms of ventilation: the positive pressure delivered by your assistant's bellows and the patient's own intrinsic breathing. The work associated with these patient-originated breaths is far more taxing, as the patient has to generate enough inspiratory force to overcome the resistance of the ventilator tubing and the endotracheal tube. This increased work can be alleviated by the addition of pressure support during the spontaneous inspiratory efforts; this mode is called *synchronized intermittent mandatory ventilation with pressure support ventilation.*

Two other forms of ventilation are more esoteric and unlikely to be initiated in the emergency department, but it would behoove the savvy emergency physician to have a certain degree of understanding of them. These methods are inverse ratio ventilation (also called *airway pressure release ventilation* [APRV]) and high-frequency oscillatory ventilation (HFOV).

Airway Pressure Release Ventilation

APRV uses prolonged periods of continuous positive airway pressure interspersed with brief periods of lower pressure. Proponents of APRV state that the prolonged periods of continuous positive airway pressure cause alveolar recruitment and thereby improve oxygenation and lung volumes without the typical alveolar stress caused by more traditional forms of mechanical ventilation. Most ventilation and CO_2 exchange occurs during the brief periods of low pressure (ie, the release phase). This strategy can be used in both spontaneously breathing and passive patients. This strategy is used most commonly for the management of ARDS and acute lung injury in the hopes of maintaining adequate oxygenation without causing iatrogenic damage to the already injured lung.[7]

High-Frequency Oscillatory Ventilation

HFOV provides an extremely high frequency of small tidal volume breaths around a high level of constant airway pressure. It is akin to instructing your assistant to attach a small engine to the bellows, which creates a propeller-driven system that delivers 30 mm Hg of continuous airway pressure. Above this pressure, the assistant is instructed to pump the bellows rapidly to deliver minuscule tidal volumes at a fast rate (3–15 Hz). Similar to APRV, this method of ventilation hopes to minimize the damage induced by mechanical ventilation by limiting the degree of alveolar distention using small tidal volumes.[8] Gas exchange is achieved by the mechanisms listed in **Table 1**.

HFOV has been used primarily in patients with ARDS but recently fell out of favor after several trials found it to be inferior to the more traditional forms of mechanical ventilation.[8]

POSTINTUBATION GOALS AND TITRATING THE VENTILATOR

The next step after selecting a mode of ventilation is verifying whether the patient is responding to it and tolerating it. This involves checking the following variables: (1) patient oxygenation, (2) degree of ventilation (ie, level of CO_2), (3) ventilator waveforms, and (4) the peak and plateau pressures.

Titrating Oxygenation

The F_{IO_2} prescribed for patients after intubation traditionally has been set at 100%, in part because of the uncertainty and acuity that often surround emergency department intubations. A level of oxygen this high should be titrated down quickly because of the harm associated with prolonged hyperoxia (levels of oxygen that are greater than needed physiologically). Several studies found that hyperoxia in certain patient populations (eg, after cardiac arrest) increases morbidity and mortality rates.[9,10] The

Table 1	
Physiologic mechanisms for gas exchange in HFOV	
Pendelluft mixing	Mixing of gas between lung units caused by impedance differences
Augmented diffusion	Gas mixing within the alveolar units
Taylor dispersion	Dispersion of molecules beyond the bulk flow front
Coaxial flow patterns	Net flow through the center of the airway on the way down, then on the outside of the airway on the way up
Cardiogenic mixing	Agitation of surrounding lung tissue with molecular diffusion

optimal oxygen level is up for debate, but it is generally considered appropriate to attain physiologic oxygen levels by titrating the FIO_2 to an oxygen saturation between 90% and 95% or a PaO_2 of 55 to 80 mm Hg.[4]

The FIO_2 level delivered to a patient is not the sole determinant of oxygenation. A patient's PaO_2 is equally affected by the proportion of alveoli participating in ventilation. By titrating the level of PEEP, you can augment the recruitment of distal alveolar tissues that were initially collapsed. Alveolar recruitment can be beneficial in patients with primary lung disorders (such as pneumonia, pulmonary edema, and ARDS) and those with otherwise healthy lungs but with portions of collapsed alveoli secondary to increased pressures external to the lung (obesity, pregnancy).[11] The use of a PEEP table (**Table 2**) allows titration in accordance with increasing the FIO_2.[12]

Titrating Ventilation

After verifying your patient's PaO_2, the next step is to verify and titrate his ventilatory effort (partial pressure of carbon dioxide, arterial), which is determined primarily by the prescribed respiratory rate (RR) and tidal volume (Vt).[13] The initial RR and Vt settings are based solely on the reason for intubation. Consideration should also be given to the use of lung-protective strategy that uses a low tidal volume (6–8 mL/kg of ideal body weight) (**Table 3**) and a respiratory rate that allows adequate time for expiration and thus avoids the phenomenon of air trapping or auto-PEEP (see later discussion).[4,13]

This low-tidal volume strategy is believed to reduce the barotrauma associated with traditional tidal volumes (ie, 8–10 mL/kg of ideal body weight), even though prospective randomized, controlled trials are lacking in non-ARDS populations.[14] If a volume mode of ventilation is chosen (ie, volume assist control), then a setting of 6 to 8 mL/kg should be chosen. If a pressure mode of ventilation is selected, then the resulting tidal volume produced from the selected pressure should also result in a tidal volume of 6 to 8 mL/kg.

The initial respiratory rate should be selected based on the primary reason for mechanical ventilation. An initial rate of 12 to 16 breaths per minute should be selected for patients who do not have ventilatory failure but were intubated for airway protection (eg, angioedema) or respiratory support (eg, severe pneumonia). Higher respiratory rates must be provided for patients requiring metabolic acidosis or CO_2 removal (eg, respiratory failure from COPD exacerbation).

Peak Pressures Versus Plateau Pressures

Let's return to our imaginary assistant and his trusty bellows. Each breath you ask him to deliver is associated with an amount of resistance he is required to overcome to pump the air into your patient's lungs. Each pump that is delivered is met with

Table 2 PEEP to FIO_2								
FIO_2	0.3	0.4	0.4	0.5	0.5	0.6	0.7	0.7	0.7
PEEP	5	5	8	8	10	10	10	12	14
FIO_2		0.8		0.9		0.9		0.9	1.0
PEEP		14		14		16		18	18–24

Data from NIH NHLBI ARDS Clinical Network Mechanical Ventilation Protocol Summary. Available at: http://www.ardsnet.org/files/ventilator_protocol_2008-07.pdf.

Table 3 Formula for ideal body weight	
Males	**Females**
IBW = 50 kg + 2.3 kg * (Height (inches) – 60)	IBW = 45.5 kg + 2.3 kg * (Height (inches) – 60)

IBW= Estimated ideal body weight in (kg).
Data from Pai MP, Paloucek FP. The origin of the "ideal" body weight equations. Ann Pharmacother 2000;34(9):1067.

opposing counter pressures arising from several sites in the bellows patient circuit — the endotracheal tube, airway secretions, the intrinsic resistance of the bronchial tree, and the elastic resistance of the alveolar tissue and the chest wall and musculature. Your assistant must overcome these pressures to deliver a successful tidal volume. The pressure that your assistant or our modern ventilators produces during inspiration is called the *driving* or *peak pressure*. The peak pressure is a combination of the resistance forces (eg, bronchoconstriction) created as airflow is moving from the bellows to the patient, plus the forces of compliance from the lung parenchyma and chest wall.[4] The peak pressure is displayed on most ventilators throughout the inspiratory cycle.

Another important pressure of which to be aware when managing ventilated patients is the plateau pressure. The plateau pressure is the compliance of the chest wall and lung parenchyma without the contribution from airway resistance. The plateau pressure is obtained by applying an inspiratory pause during a mechanical breath that will result in no airflow between the ventilator and patient.

The peak and plateau pressures can be used clinically to assess both the resistive and compliant forces of the patient–ventilator circuit. If the plateau and peak pressures are both elevated, the patient might have a problem with compliance (eg, pneumothorax, ARDS). A high peak pressure with a normal or low plateau pressure is likely caused by access resistance in the ventilator circuit. This can be extrinsic resistance (eg, kinked or small endotracheal tube) or intrinsic (eg, asthma, COPD). **Table 4** presents a more complete differential diagnosis for peak and plateau pressures.

DAMAGE CONTROL VENTILATION

Significant energy has been devoted to investigating the efficacy of each mode of ventilation, but no single strategy has distinguished itself as superior. Dogmatic support for one mode over the other is not supported by the literature.[15,16] A more

Table 4 Peak and plateau pressures	
Peak = Plateau (Problem of Compliance)	**Peak > Plateau (Problem of Resistance)**
ARDS	Bronchoconstriction (eg, COPD/asthma)
Pneumothorax	Kinked endotracheal tube
Pulmonary edema	Mucus in endotracheal tube
Pleural effusion	Mucus in bronchi
Atelectasis	Small diameter endotracheal tube
Main stem intubation	
External compression of chest (eg, supine position in obese patient)	

practical approach is to select the mode of ventilation with which you are most comfortable and use the strategies discussed in the following section to guide ventilator management.

Several considerations must be taken into consideration when determining the mode of ventilation used in the emergency department, most notably that positive-pressure ventilation is harmful to our patients.[17–19] In addition to being traumatic and painful, it disrupts almost all the body's natural physiologic processes. In this section, we discuss the harmful effects of positive-pressure ventilation and how to ameliorate them.

The first and most apparent harm is the effect of positive-pressure ventilation on the patient's cardiac output. Our usual negative pressure state augments the circulatory system. During spontaneous inhalation, a negative pressure is generated in the thoracic cavity, leading to an increase in the pressure gradient between the venous system and the right ventricle. This increase augments venous return and, in turn, cardiac output. Conversely, when we supplement a patient's ventilatory effort by providing positive-pressure ventilation, we are creating positive pressures in the thoracic cavity. This, of course, has exactly the opposite effect on venous return. In a healthy subject with adequate volume reserve and an intact autonomic response, such perturbation typically goes unnoticed. But this subject is rarely the one we need to intubate in the emergency department. Patients who need to be intubated are incredibly sick, severely volume depleted, and typically have some degree of autonomic dysfunction. Therefore, it is not unusual for patients who undergo intubation and subsequent ventilation to display episodes of hypotension and even cardiac arrest.[20] Studies have found that 22% of patients who are intubated in the emergency department experienced some degree of hypotension and that 4.2% experience cardiac arrest.[21,22] Disruption of the circulatory system should be anticipated, and adequate fluid and vasopressor support should be provided before intubation and during the early period of mechanical ventilation.

The second consideration is the direct iatrogenic effect of mechanical ventilation on the lung parenchyma, which emerges days after patients have left our care in the emergency department. The concept of lung-protective ventilation was born out of the management of patients with ARDS.[23,24] In the past, these patients were commonly exposed to high tidal volumes and F_{IO_2} levels in an attempt to correct their metabolic disturbances. Although there was some awareness that such strategies worsened lung injury, the pervasive thought was that maintaining hemostasis was more important than preventing lung injury. This assumption was challenged by the ARDSNet protocol. The authors of that protocol claimed that attempts to correct metabolic and ventilatory abnormalities damaged the lungs and led to worse downstream outcomes. These investigators proposed that a lung-protective strategy should be used instead, accepting some degree of hypoxia and acidosis to preserve lung function. The authors theorized that this strategy would not only reduce lung injury but also decrease the mortality rate.[23,24] Subsequent studies found that lung-protective ventilation does indeed decrease rates of lung injury and ARDS when initiated in the emergency department.[25] We should strive to apply a low tidal volume strategy (6–8 mL/kg) for most patients who undergo mechanical ventilation in the emergency department. Furthermore, we must resist the urge to overcorrect these patients in the hopes of making their numbers look better without deriving any true clinical benefit. We should limit our oxygenation and ventilation goals to Pa_{O_2} levels of 55 to 80 mm Hg and pH >7.3. Further correction is likely to yield more harm than benefit.[25]

The third concept of damage control ventilation is prophylactically protecting against breath stacking (auto-PEEP). As discussed earlier, breath stacking occurs when the ventilator initiates a breath before the patient is fully able to exhale the prior inhalation. This process leads to a certain volume of gas being trapped in the lung with each exhalation. As this volume grows, it becomes large enough to hyperdistend the lungs, causing parenchymal damage, decreasing venous return, and potentially resulting in pneumothorax. To prevent these complications, a sufficiently slow RR, low Vt, and high inspiratory flow time should be used.[26] These settings can cause a state of hypoventilation, but, similar to lung-protective ventilation, these prophylactic measures anticipate the patient becoming acidotic, with the knowledge that breath stacking leads to greater downstream harm than persistent mild respiratory acidosis.[25]

The final consideration is the ventilation of patients with severe metabolic acidosis, who are typically breathing at a high rate to compensate for their metabolic derangement. After intubation, we should attempt to match their preintubated intrinsic respiratory rate so as not to considerably exacerbate their acidosis by eliminating their respiratory drive. Of course, this approach cannot be universal; the degree of extrinsic mechanical compensation will vary depending on the cause of the patient's acidosis. For example, a young healthy patient with diabetic ketoacidosis often functions well in severely acidotic states with little physiologic perturbation. On the other hand, a critically ill patient with salicylate poisoning will become severely compromised with even slight decreases in the pH, because the amount of toxin in its uncharged form (capable of crossing the blood–brain barrier) increases dramatically in an acidotic environment.[26]

TROUBLESHOOTING THE VENTILATOR

Even though we do our best to anticipate the problems associated with mechanical ventilation, challenges still arise. Therefore, it is important to have an efficient and comprehensive strategy for diagnosing and managing each unique situation. Situations requiring troubleshooting can be divided into 2 categories: those involving patients facing hemodynamic and ventilator collapse and others involving hemodynamically stable patients whose ventilator malfunctions.

The latter is obviously far less serious and allows time for evaluation and diagnosis of the problem. In such cases, we can evaluate the patient's respiratory status, including oxygenation, ventilation, waveform analysis, and peak and plateau pressures. Specific questions should focus on hypoxia, hypoventilation, air hunger, auto-PEEP, pneumothoraxes, and compliance and resistance problems.[27]

The crashing ventilated patient presents a more urgent and immediate scenario. In these cases, we must rapidly assess, diagnose, and treat any correctable issue that is or might cause these patients to decompensate.[27] A helpful mnemonic to guide this assessment is DOPES: displaced tube/endotracheal cuff, obstructed tube, pneumothorax, equipment malfunction, and stacking breaths. These are the 5 common and correctable causes of severe ventilatory dysfunction. To correct each of these

Table 5 DOPES and DOTTS mnemonic	
Causes of Hemodynamic Instability	Empiric Treatment for Ventilator-Induced Hemodynamic Instability
Displaced endotracheal tube	Disconnect from the ventilator
Obstructed endotracheal tube	Oxygen, 100% on the BVM
Pneumothorax	Tube position
Equipment failure	Tweak the ventilator
Stacking breaths	Sonographic evaluation for pneumothorax

problems, the mnemonic DOTTS can be used: disconnect the patient from the ventilator, O_2 100% using the BVM, tube position, tweak the ventilator, sonographically evaluate for pneumothorax (**Table 5**).

SUMMARY

Mechanical ventilation is a commonly used but sometimes poorly understood modality in the emergency department. Traditionally, emergency physicians have left the nuances of this therapy to the respiratory therapists and critical care physicians. In the modern-day emergency department, in which patients remain under our care for longer periods, we must become comfortable with treating ventilated patients for an extended time. Therefore, it is necessary that we understand how to initiate, titrate, and treat patients on a mechanical ventilator. This skill set includes the ability to adapt ventilatory strategies for specific patients an understanding of the potential harms of mechanical ventilation, and the ability to take action to reduce their incidence.

REFERENCES

1. Pierson DJ. Noninvasive positive pressure ventilation: history and terminology. Respir Care 1997;42:370–9.
2. Lawrence G. Tools of the trade: tobacco smoke enemas. Lancet 2002;359:1442.
3. Colice GL. Historical perspective on the development of mechanical ventilation. In: Tobin MJ, editor. Principles and practice of mechanical ventilation. New York: McGraw-Hill; 1994. p. 1–35.
4. Owens W. The ventilator book. First Draught Press; 2012.
5. Hamed Hala MF, Ibrahim HG, Khater YH, et al. Ventilation and ventilators in the ICU: what every intensivist must know. Curr Anaesth Crit Care 2006;17:77–83.
6. Przybysz, Heffner. Early treatment of severe ARDS, in press.
7. Daoud EG. Airway pressure release ventilation. Ann Thorac Med 2007;2:176–9.
8. Ferguson ND, Cook DJ, Guyatt GH, et al. High-frequency oscillation in early acute respiratory distress syndrome. N Engl J Med 2013;368:795–805.
9. Helmerhorst H, Roos-Blom MJ, van Westerloo DJ, et al. Association Between Arterial Hyperoxia and Outcome in Subsets of Critical Illness: A Systematic Review, Metaanalysis, and Meta-Regression of Cohort Studies. Crit Care Med 2015;43(7):1508–19.
10. Damiani E, Adrario E, Girardis M, et al. Arterial hyperoxia and mortality in critically ill patients: a systematic review and meta-analysis. Crit Care 2014;18(6):711.
11. Lemyze M. Effects of sitting position and applied positive end-expiratory pressure on respiratory mechanics of critically ill obese patients receiving mechanical ventilation. Crit Care Med 2013;41:2592–9.
12. Brower RG, Lanken PN, MacIntyre N, et al. Higher versus lower positive end-expiratory pressures in patients with the acute respiratory distress syndrome. N Engl J Med 2004;351:327–36.
13. Marino P. The ICU book. Philadelphia: Lippincott, Williams & Wilkins; 2014.
14. Serpa Neto A, Naqtzaam L, Schultz MJ. Ventilation with lower tidal volumes for critically ill patients without the acute respiratory distress syndrome: a systematic translational review and meta-analysis. Curr Opin Crit Care 2014;20:25–32.
15. Schultz MJ, Haitsma JJ, Slutsky AS, et al. What tidal volumes should be used in patients without acute lung injury? Anesthesiology 2007;106:1226–31.
16. Rittayamai N, Katsios CM, Beloncle F, et al. Pressure-controlled versus volume-controlled ventilation in acute respiratory failure: a physiology-based narrative and systematic review. Chest 2015;148(2):340–55.

17. Dreyfuss D, Saumon G. Ventilator-induced lung injury: lessons from experimental studies. Am J Respir Crit Care Med 1998;157:294–323.
18. Carney D, DiRocco J, Nieman G. Dynamic alveolar mechanics and ventilator-induced lung injury. Crit Care Med 2005;33:S122–8.
19. Plotz FB, Slutsky AS, van Vught AJ, et al. Ventilator-induced lung injury and multiple system organ failure: a critical review of facts and hypotheses. Intensive Care Med 2004;30:1865–72.
20. Jaber S, Amraoui J, Lefrant JY, et al. Clinical practice and risk factors for immediate complications of endotracheal intubation in the intensive care unit: a prospective, multiple-center study. Crit Care Med 2006;34:2355–61.
21. Heffner AC, Swords DS, Neale MN, et al. Incidence and factors associated with cardiac arrest complicating emergency airway management. Resuscitation 2013; 84:1500–4.
22. Heffner AC, Swords DS, Nussbaum ML, et al. Predictors of the complication of postintubation hypotension during emergency airway management. J Crit Care 2012;27:587–93.
23. Ventilation with lower tidal volumes as compared with traditional tidal volumes for acute lung injury and the acute respiratory distress syndrome: the Acute Respiratory Distress Syndrome Network. N Engl J Med 2000;342:1301–8.
24. Amato MB, Barbas CS, Medeiros DM, et al. Effect of a protective-ventilation strategy on mortality in the acute respiratory distress syndrome. N Engl J Med 1998; 338:347–54.
25. Determann RM, Royakkers A, Wolthuis EK, et al. Ventilation with lower tidal volumes as compared with conventional tidal volumes for patients without acute lung injury: a preventive randomized controlled trial. Crit Care 2010;14(1):R1.
26. Stolbach AI, Hoffman RS, Nelson LS. Mechanical ventilation was associated with acidemia in a case series of salicylate-poisoned patients. Acad Emerg Med 2008;15:866–9.
27. Santanilla JI. The crashing ventilated patient. In: Winters ME, et al, editors. Emergency Department resuscitation of the critically ill. Dallas (TX): American College of Emergency Physicians; 2011. p. 15–24.

Pediatric Respiratory Emergencies

Amber M. Richards, MD

KEYWORDS

- Pediatric respiratory emergency • Foreign body aspiration • Asthma • Epiglottitis
- Bronchiolitis • Pneumonia

KEY POINTS

- Children with respiratory complaints commonly present to the ED and it is imperative that physicians be able to promptly recognize and treat these disease processes.
- Maintain a high level of suspicion for foreign body aspiration in patients with good history even when presenting with normal examination.
- Provide supportive management in epiglottitis without increasing anxiety or agitation and involve consultants early.
- Bronchiolitis treatment recommendations have changed based on current AAP guidelines. Supportive care is the mainstay of current bronchiolitis therapy.

Respiratory emergencies are 1 of the most common reasons parents seek evaluation for the their children in the emergency department (ED) each year, and respiratory failure is the most common cause of cardiopulmonary arrest in pediatric patients. Whereas many respiratory illnesses are mild and self-limiting, others are life threatening and require prompt diagnosis and management. Therefore, it is imperative that emergency clinicians be able to promptly recognize and manage these illnesses. This article reviews ED diagnosis and management of foreign body aspiration, asthma exacerbation, epiglottitis, bronchiolitis, community-acquired pneumonia, and pertussis.

NONINFECTIOUS EMERGENCIES
Foreign Body Aspiration

Epidemiology

Although recognition and management has improved, foreign body aspiration (FBA) remains common in children. FBA can occur in children of all ages, although most occurrences are in children younger than 4 years, with a peak incidence between the first and second birthdays.[1] White and colleagues[2] reviewed FBA cases from

Disclosure: The authors have nothing to disclose.
Department of Emergency Medicine, Maine Medical Center, Tufts University School of Medicine, 22 Bramhall Street, Portland, ME 04103, USA
E-mail address: richaa2@mmc.org

Emerg Med Clin N Am 34 (2016) 77–96
http://dx.doi.org/10.1016/j.emc.2015.08.006
emed.theclinics.com
0733-8627/16/$ – see front matter © 2016 Elsevier Inc. All rights reserved.

1955 to 1960 and compared these with FBA cases from 1999 to 2003. Comparison revealed similarities in the types of aspirated foreign bodies. Organic foreign bodies were the most common (**Fig. 1**).[3,4] The type of foreign body aspirated should raise concern about different airway problems (**Box 1**).

Clinical presentation

It is important to maintain a high degree of suspicion for FBA. A large number of patients presenting with a good history and normal examination were found to have FBA.[5] Conversely, one should also be concerned if there is a poor history but good examination for FBA because approximately half of cases occur without a choking event having been witnessed.[6,7] Clinical symptoms and signs vary based on the location of the foreign body and the degree of obstruction (**Box 2**).

One complicating factor is that the clinical presentation may change over time as a result of movement of the foreign body within the respiratory tract. It is also important to remember that an ingested foreign body lodged in the upper thorax may cause compression or local inflammation leading to respiratory distress that is indistinguishable from an aspirated foreign body.

Evaluation

Neck and chest radiographs, including posteroanterior (PA) and lateral views, should be obtained to evaluate for the presence of a foreign body. Radiopaque foreign bodies are easily visualized on radiographs, whereas radiolucent foreign bodies pose a greater challenge. If a foreign body is not radiopaque, the evaluator should look for secondary signs of FBA such as overinflation, opacification, or atelectasis of the distal lung (**Fig. 2**).

Additional radiography views such as inspiratory and expiratory views or lateral decubitus views may be obtained[8] (**Fig. 3**). Fluoroscopy is also beneficial in the diagnosis of FBA, particularly in young patients who cannot cooperate with inspiratory and expiratory views. Recent studies investigated the use of virtual bronchoscopy (computerized tomography [CT]) as a noninvasive alternative to diagnose and localize aspirated foreign bodies (**Fig. 4**). When obstructive pathology is depicted with virtual bronchoscopy, a therapeutic bronchoscopy should be performed; however, in cases where no obstructive pathology is detected, proceeding to rigid bronchoscopy might not be clinically useful.[9]

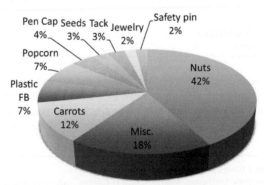

Fig. 1. Foreign body type. (*Data from* Tan HK, Brown K, McGill T, et al. Airway foreign bodies (FB): a 10-year review. Int J Pediatr Otorhinolaryngol 2000;56(2):91–9; and Hsu, W, Sheen TS, Lin CD, et al. Clinical experiences of removing foreign bodies in the airway and esophagus with a rigid endoscope: a series of 3217 cases from 1970 to 1996. Otolaryngol Head Neck Surg 2000;122(3):450–4.)

Box 1
Types of aspirated foreign bodies and resulting airway issues

- Inorganic material such as glass or metal
  - Little tissue inflammation
  - Direct airway injury if sharp
- Organic material such as nuts
  - Significant inflammation
  - Formation of granulation tissue
- Button battery
  - Inflammation
  - Ulceration
  - Burns/necrosis
- Medications
  - Inflammation
  - Ulceration

Management

A child who has partial airway obstruction and is breathing spontaneously should be kept calm and given supplemental oxygen as needed. If the child is in extremis or respiratory arrest occurs, immediate airway management should be performed. If respiratory arrest does occur and a foreign body is visible above the vocal cords during laryngoscopy, an attempt should be made to extract it with Magill forceps. If the foreign body is below the vocal cords, it is reasonable to attempt to push the foreign body more distally to reestablish a patent airway. This may allow for rescue oxygenation and ventilation while preparing for more definitive management.

A patient with a highly suggestive clinical picture should undergo diagnostic and therapeutic endoscopy, even if imaging is negative.[6,7,10] Depending on the practice at individual hospitals, this will include assistance from otolaryngology, pediatric pulmonology, or pediatric surgery departments. Rigid bronchoscopy has been the mainstay of retrieval in the past; however, multiple recent investigations have evaluated the use of flexible bronchoscopy for foreign body retrieval. These studies have shown that, in cases of suspected FBA, rigid bronchoscopy should be performed when presentation includes asphyxia, radiopaque foreign body on imaging, unilateral decreased breath sounds, localized wheezing on examination, or obstructive radiological emphysema or atelectasis.[11,12] In all other cases, flexible bronchoscopy or virtual bronchoscopy may be performed first for diagnostic purposes.[11,12] If the obstruction cannot be removed by flexible bronchoscopy, the patient may require rigid

---

Box 2
Clinical signs and symptoms of foreign body aspiration

- Upper airway foreign body
  - Cough
  - Stridor
  - Respiratory or cardiopulmonary arrest
- Lower airway foreign body
  - Cough
  - Wheezing
  - Retractions/accessory muscle use
  - Decreased breath sounds

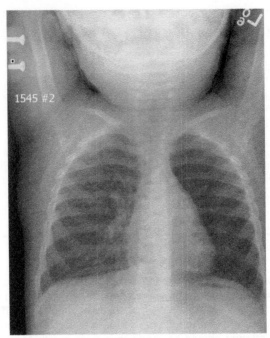

Fig. 2. Hyperinflation of left lower lung caused by aspirated peanut husk in a 15-month-old patient.

bronchoscopy. Thus, flexible bronchoscopy should be performed in a setting where back-up rigid bronchoscopy is available.[11] Although adults may tolerate bronchoscopy under moderate sedation, it is optimal for pediatric bronchoscopy to be performed in an operating room for improved airway control and optimal patient comfort (**Fig. 5**).[11,12]

Asthma

Epidemiology

Asthma is 1 of the most common serious chronic diseases affecting children. It is a chronic inflammatory process affecting the lower airways. This chronic inflammation causes episodic wheezing, cough, and shortness of breath. Children between the ages of 5 and 17 years affected by asthma account for one-third of all asthma-related ED visits. The annual health care cost including direct and indirect expenses and lost productivity costs amounts to a total yearly sum of $20.7 billion. Asthma alone accounts for 14.4 million missed school days per year.[13]

Clinical presentation

The clinical presentation of patients with an acute asthma exacerbation varies depending on the baseline severity of the asthma, as well as the severity of the current episode. Clinicians should evaluate for triggers causing the acute exacerbation to address any treatable cause in addition to managing the patient's symptoms (**Box 3**).

Patients with an acute exacerbation may present complaining of wheezing, cough, shortness of breath, or chest tightness. Physical examination findings vary depending on whether a patient is presenting with mild, moderate, or severe exacerbation (**Box 4**).

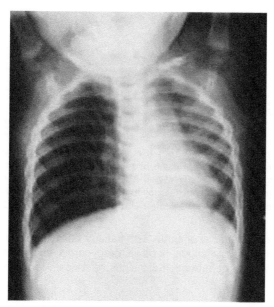

Fig. 3. Expiratory view with hyperexpansion and hyperlucency in the right lung caused by a foreign body in the right mainstem. Mediastinal shift toward the left lung. Inspiratory: moderate hyperlucency and hyperexpansion of the right hemithorax. A mild deviation of the mediastinum toward the left chest is noted. Expiratory: hyperlucency and hyperexpansion of the right hemithorax. A greater mediastinal shift is noted toward the left lung field.

Investigation should include a thorough history of previous exacerbations, including rapidity of onset, number of episodes in the last year, need for hospitalization, and any previous intubations. Patients with persistent asthmatic symptoms and previous severe exacerbations are more likely to experience recurrent severe asthma exacerbations.[14]

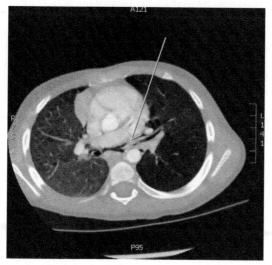

Fig. 4. Obstructing peanut husk in the left mainstem bronchus in a 15-month-old patient. *Arrow* pointing to obstructing peanut husk.

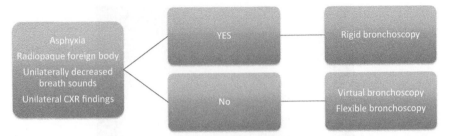

Fig. 5. Aspirated Foreign Body Algorithm. (*Data from* Zerella JT, Dimler M, McGill LC, et al. Foreign body aspiration in children: value of radiography and complications of bronchoscopy. J Pediatr Surg 1998;33(11):1651–4; and Righini CA, Morel N, Karkas A, et al. What is the diagnostic value of flexible bronchoscopy in the initial investigation of children with suspected foreign body aspiration? Int J Pediatr Otorhinolaryngol 2007;71:1383–90.)

During severe exacerbations or status asthmaticus, children may become confused and somnolent. Respiratory fatigue, hypoxia, bradycardia, and absence of wheezing caused by severe airway obstruction are signs of concern for imminent respiratory arrest.

Evaluation

Pulse oximetry should be measured in all children presenting with an asthma exacerbation and should be continuously monitored in those with moderate to severe exacerbations.

Laboratory testing and imaging are not mandatory for the diagnosis and management of an acute asthma exacerbation. However, depending on preceding history, testing may be indicated to evaluate for an asthma trigger, rule out an alternate condition, or evaluate for complications associated with asthma.

Peak flow testing before and after bronchodilator therapy is helpful for assessing response to therapy in older children but is difficult to obtain in younger or uncooperative children. Obtaining an arterial blood gas measurement in severe exacerbations and status asthmaticus may be useful to assess for respiratory function and response to therapy.

Several clinical assessment tools exist, including the Pulmonary Index, Pulmonary Score, Pediatric Asthma Severity Score (PASS), and Pediatric Respiratory Assessment Measure (PRAM). The PASS and PRAM scores included preschool-age children in their derivation and both have shown the ability to predict prolonged ED stay or admission. They are useful tools in the evaluation of asthma exacerbations.[15–18]

Box 3
Asthma triggers

- Infections (viral or bacterial)
- Environmental allergens
- Changes in weather
- Irritants (smoke exposure, vapors)
- Emotional stressors
- Exercise
- Food

Box 4
Physical examination findings for acute exacerbation

- Wheezing
- Diminished breath sounds
- Cough
- Increased respiratory rate
- Accessory muscle use
- Retractions
- Tachycardia
- Dyspnea with speaking

Management

Patients should be rapidly assessed, have early initiation of management, and frequent reassessment while in the ED. Oxygen should be administered if hypoxemia is present.

Short-acting β-agonist medications are first-line therapy for treating bronchospasm in acute asthma exacerbations. They may be administered continuously via nebulizer or intermittently via metered dose inhaler (MDI) with spacer. In mild to moderate asthma, treatment with an MDI is equivalent to nebulizer administration.[19–23] Bronchodilators given by MDI have also been shown to be more cost effective compared with nebulization.[24,25] Patient cooperation may be a factor in the choice of nebulizer or MDI treatment. More severe exacerbations may benefit from continuous medication administration via nebulizer. Ipratropium bromide (Atrovent), when combined with short-acting β-agonists, has proved beneficial in moderate to severe exacerbations[26,27]; it causes smooth muscle relaxation through muscarinic acetylcholine receptor blockade, resulting in bronchodilation. Ipratropium bromide may be administered by intermittent MDI or in combined nebulizer treatment with a β-agonist.[26,27]

Early ED treatment with systemic corticosteroids has been shown to decrease admission rates and length of hospital stay and should be considered in all asthma exacerbations.[28–31] Initiation of corticosteroid treatment in triage has proved beneficial.[32] Efficacy of oral versus parenteral administration is equivalent,[33] therefore systemic corticosteroids should be administered orally unless the patient is not tolerating administration by mouth. Prednisone or prednisolone over 3 to 5 days has been the standard therapy. However, research has demonstrated that a single dose or a 2-day course of dexamethasone is as effective and has improved tolerance when considering rates of nausea and vomiting.[34–40] Inhaled corticosteroids do not replace the need for systemic corticosteroids in acute asthma exacerbations[41,42] (**Table 1**).

In severe or refractory asthma exacerbations, additional therapies may be necessary. Magnesium sulfate has been shown to cause bronchodilation and is safe and well tolerated. It has not been shown to have any effect in mild to moderate

---

Table 1
Systemic corticosteroids dosing

Prednisone/prednisolone	1–2 mg/kg po daily for 3–5 d (maximum dose 60 mg/d)
Dexamethasone	0.6 mg/kg po daily for 1–2 d
	0.6 mg/kg IV/IM for 1 dose (maximum dose 16 mg/d)

exacerbations, but research has demonstrated that its use results in decreased admission rates in severe asthma exacerbations.[43] A single intravenous dose of magnesium sulfate of 25 to 75 mg/kg not exceeding 2 g may be given over 2 hours. Evidence is conflicting regarding the benefits of Heliox, a blend of helium and oxygen, in asthma exacerbations.[44–51] Lack of portability may cause a delay in administration thus limiting its use in the ED. For intubated patients on mechanical ventilation, Heliox may assist in lowering peak inspiratory pressure and improving blood gas pH and partial pressure CO_2.[47]

In status asthmaticus and imminent respiratory failure, a trial of noninvasive positive-pressure ventilation (NPPV) may be used in an attempt to avoid intubation. However, if the patient is unable to tolerate NPPV or continues to deteriorate, endotracheal intubation will be necessary. If intubation is necessary, appropriate ventilator management is of utmost importance. Permissive hypercapnea, with P_{CO_2} up to 70 mm Hg, has been shown to be beneficial.[52] Ventilator settings should be adjusted to provide prolonged expiratory time allowing for complete exhalation to avoid barotrauma and other complications.[50,52,53]

Indications for admission

- Respiratory distress (grunting, nasal flaring, retractions)
- Hypoxia
- Little or no response to therapy
- Social concerns (no access to follow-up, transport, and so forth)

INFECTIOUS EMERGENCIES
Epiglottitis

Epidemiology
Epiglottitis is a severe potentially life-threatening condition in which there is acute inflammation of the epiglottis and surrounding tissues. Inflammation and edema lead to progressive airway obstruction and can cause respiratory arrest. It is most often caused by bacterial infection but can also occur as a result of thermal or inhalational injury or local trauma.[54] Before the advent of the Haemophilus influenza type B (Hib) vaccine, Haemophilus influenzae caused almost all pediatric cases of epiglottitis, with a peak incidence in children between 2 and 4 years old. Since the development and administration of this vaccine, epiglottitis has become less common with an incidence of 1.3 cases per 100,000 children.[55,56] Currently, the most common causes of epiglottitis are group A beta-hemolytic streptococcus, Streptococcus pneumonia, Klebsiella sp, and Staphyloccocus aureus.[57] The shift in pathogens indicates need for adjustment of antibiotic therapy. As a result of vaccination against Hib and alternative pathogens causing epiglottitis, fewer cases have been seen in children of all ages as well as in adults.[57]

Clinical presentation
The typical presentation for epiglottitis includes abrupt onset of symptoms including high fever, sore throat, irritability, drooling caused by dysphagia, muffled voice, and progressive respiratory distress. Onset occurs rapidly without prodromal symptoms. Children appear toxic and the respiratory symptoms may contribute to a high level of anxiety. Because of airway obstruction, patients may prefer resting in the tripod position (ie, leaning forward with jaw protrusion). Cyanosis and stridor may be present late in the course or in severe cases and are of concern because of possible respiratory failure.

Evaluation
The most important aspect of evaluation in children with suspected epiglottitis is to keep the patient calm to avoid worsening respiratory compromise. If possible,

evaluation of the oropharynx is beneficial because the tip of an enlarged erythematous epiglottis may be visualized or an alternate condition such as peritonsillar abscess may be seen. However, use of a tongue depressor or other equipment that may agitate the patient is discouraged. Laboratory studies are unlikely to be helpful in the acute management of epiglottitis and intravenous placement or venipuncture should be postponed until the airway is stable. Radiography may be helpful in evaluation but should only be performed if it does not distress the patient. The classic finding for epiglottitis on lateral neck radiographs is the "thumbprint sign" caused by the thickened and enlarged epiglottis. The absence of this sign does not rule out epiglottitis. Alternatively, imaging may help diagnose a foreign body, retropharyngeal abscess, or other cause of respiratory distress. CT may be helpful in diagnosis, but should only be performed in mild cases where lying supine does not cause airway compromise or patient distress. Ultimately, diagnosis requires direct visualization of the epiglottis using laryngoscopy.

Management
Airway management is of utmost importance in epiglottitis and care should be taken to avoid procedures that increase the child's anxiety until after their airway is secured. Early otolaryngology and anesthesiology consultation is important because direct laryngoscopy is definitive for diagnosis, and airway management in a controlled setting is optimal. Airway management resources and tools should be readily available for the duration of time the child is present in the ED. If respiratory failure occurs while in the ED, airway management including intubation should be carried out. Because of airway inflammation, it is important to remember that an endotracheal tube smaller than that calculated according to age may be needed.[58]

Once the airway is secure, appropriate antibiotic treatment should be initiated (**Box 5**).

Although no randomized control trials have evaluated the use of steroids in the epiglottitis, steroids are commonly used to decrease inflammation in the airway.

Bronchiolitis

Epidemiology
Bronchiolitis is a viral infection affecting the lower respiratory tract in children. It is characterized by acute inflammation of the lower airways and increased mucous production.[59] Numerous viruses can cause bronchiolitis including, but not limited to, respiratory syncytial virus (RSV), human rhinovirus, human metapneumovirus, influenza,

---

Box 5
Antibiotic coverage for epiglottitis

Antibiotics for epiglottitis

- Ampicillin/sulbactam
- Cefotaxime
- Ceftriaxone
- Clindamycin[a]

If MRSA is suspected add

- Vancomycin

  [a] Alternative if penicillin or cephalosporin allergy.

and adenovirus. Although bronchiolitis may occur in children of all ages, the most severe presentations occur in children under 2 years as their smaller airways do not tolerate mucosal edema (**Box 6**). Bronchiolitis is the most common cause of infant hospitalizations in the first year of life, accounting for approximately 100,000 admissions in the United States annually at an estimated cost of $1.73 billion.[60] Hall and colleagues[61] performed a prospective analysis of RSV hospitalizations and found that the hospitalization rate was 5.2 per 1000 children less than 2 years of age, with the highest rate of hospitalization occurring among infants between 30 and 60 days of age.

Clinical presentation

The goal during the history and physical examination is to distinguish patients with viral bronchiolitis from those with other diagnoses and to determine the severity of illness. Signs and symptoms of bronchiolitis include symptoms of upper respiratory infection such as rhinorrhea and cough, fever, wheezing, respiratory distress, poor feeding, and apnea. Examination findings vary from mild to severe. Patients may present with tachypnea, nasal flaring, grunting, cyanosis, accessory muscle use, retractions, and diffuse crackles on auscultation.

Evaluation

Bronchiolitis is a clinical diagnosis based on history and physical examination. No routine laboratory testing or imaging is recommended.[59] In instances where another diagnosis is considered, laboratory tests and imaging may be necessary to evaluate for an alternative diagnosis. RSV testing is not routinely recommended and is indicated for epidemiologic purposes only.[59] Studies have shown that children with suspected viral lower respiratory infection who had radiography performed were more likely to receive antibiotics without change in outcome.[62,63] Radiography should be reserved for patients in whom alternative or complicating diagnoses are suspected.[62,63]

Management

Based on literature review and the new American Academy of Pediatrics (AAP) Bronchiolitis Guideline, many treatments previously used in bronchiolitis are no longer recommended (**Box 7**).[59]

In addition, albuterol is not recommended for isolated bronchiolitis.[59] However, if there is evidence of bronchospasm or if the patient has a history of asthma, a trial of albuterol should be considered. If there is no response after the initial trial of albuterol, it should be discontinued.[59] Maintenance of hydration and nutrition is important

---

Box 6
Risk factors for severe bronchiolitis

- Age less than 12 weeks
- Prematurity
- Cardiac disease
- Pulmonary disease
- Immunodeficiency

Data from Subcommittee on Bronchiolitis. Clinical practice guideline: the diagnosis, management, and prevention or bronchiolitis. Pediatrics 2014;134:e1474–502; and Ricart S, Marcos MA, Sarda M, et al. Clinical risk factors are more relevant than respiratory viruses in predicting bronchiolitis severity. Pediatr Pulmonol 2013;48(5):456–63.

> **Box 7**
> **Treatments not indicated for bronchiolitis**
>
> - Antihistamines
> - Decongestants
> - Racemic epinephrine
> - Steroids
> - Hypertonic saline
> - Antibiotics
> - Cool mist
> - Chest physiotherapy
> - Deep suctioning

in bronchiolitis management. Oral hydration and nutrition are preferable; however, intravenous fluids may be required when significant dehydration is present or if respiratory distress prevents the child hydrating orally. Supplemental oxygen should be used to maintain oxygen saturations greater than 90%.[59] Variability in clinical appearance may necessitate serial examinations or admission for observation.

Indications for admission[59]

- Respiratory distress (grunting, nasal flaring, retractions)
- Hypoxia
- Difficulty feeding or maintaining hydration
- Social concerns (no access to follow-up, transport, and so forth)

Pneumonia

Epidemiology

Community-acquired pneumonia (CAP) is a common pediatric respiratory infection and a leading cause of annual morbidity and mortality. Although CAP can occur at any age, it is more common in younger children. Pneumonia accounts for 13% of all infectious illnesses in infants younger than 2 years.[64] Widespread use of the heptavalent pneumococcal vaccine has reduced the incidence of pneumonia among children younger than 5 years.[65] As use of the 13-valent conjugated pneumococcal vaccine becomes prevalent, the overall rates of pneumonia are anticipated to drop further. Causative organisms of CAP vary by patient age[66–69] (**Table 2**).

Clinical presentation

Neonates with pneumonia present with fever, irritability, poor feeding, hypoxemia, or respiratory distress, but rarely cough. Beyond the neonatal period, infants with CAP may present with cough in addition to the above symptoms. Toddlers and older children typically present with fever, upper respiratory congestion, and cough. It should be noted that fever is common with bacterial pneumonia; however, if the causative agent is viral, fever may be absent. Decreased activity, decreased appetite and oral intake, headache, and vague abdominal pain may also be present in children with pneumonia. Physical examination may be nonspecific and vary based on age and infectious organism involved. Visual inspection of the degree of respiratory effort and accessory muscle use should be performed to assess for the presence and severity of respiratory distress (**Box 8**).

Table 2	
Causative organisms of community-acquired pneumonia	
Age	**Organism**
Birth–3 wk	Group B *Streptococcus*[a]
	Gram-negative bacteria[a]
	Listeria monocytogenes
3 wk–3 mo	*Streptococcus pneumoniae*
3 mo–preschool age	Viral
	S pneumoniae[b]
	Mycomplasma pneumoniae
	Haemophilus influenzae type B
	Staphylococcus aureus
School aged and adolescents	*M pneumoniae*
	S pneumoniae
	Viral

[a] Mirror pathogens responsible for neonatal sepsis.
[b] Most prominent bacterial cause in this age range.
Data from Refs.[66–69]

Auscultation is important in the evaluation of pneumonia but often difficult in infants and young children because of agitation or crying. The presence of crackles or rales is a classic indication for pneumonia, although focal crackles are neither sensitive nor specific for the diagnosis of pneumonia.[70–72] The absence of abnormal breath sounds on auscultation does not rule out the diagnosis of pneumonia. Rales and rhonchi are observed much less frequently in infants with pneumonia than in older individuals. Asymmetric breath sounds, such as focal wheezing or decreased breath sounds in 1 lung field, are suggestive of pneumonia. Atypical bacterial pneumonia and viral pneumonia may present with more diffuse crackles or wheezing.

Evaluation

Pulse oximetry should be performed in all children with respiratory symptoms to evaluate for hypoxemia. The presence of hypoxemia should guide decisions regarding

Box 8
Signs of respiratory distress
• Tachypnea (breaths/min)[a]
○ Age 0 to 2 months greater than 60
○ Age 2 to 12 months greater than 50
○ Age 1 to 5 years greater than 40
○ Age greater than 5 years greater than 20
• Retractions (suprasternal, intercostal, subcostal)
• Grunting
• Nasal flaring
• Lethargy/altered mental status
• Apnea
• Pulse oximetry measuring less than 90%
[a] Adapted from World Health Organization criteria.

further diagnostic testing and patient disposition.[73] Routine measurement of the complete blood cell count is not necessary in children with suspected CAP who may be managed in the outpatient setting. However, in those with more serious disease, it may provide useful information when combined with clinical examination and other laboratory and imaging studies. Acute-phase reactants, such as erythrocyte sedimentation rate, C-reactive protein, or serum procalcitonin concentration, cannot be used as the sole determinant to distinguish between viral and bacterial causes. They do not provide additional value in well-appearing children with CAP receiving outpatient management. Acute-phase reactants may provide helpful information regarding response to therapy in patients with severe disease requiring hospitalization.[73] Blood cultures should not be routinely performed in nontoxic children with CAP. They should be obtained in patients who appear toxic or who fail to demonstrate clinical improvement despite appropriate therapy.[73] Several studies have shown that clinical diagnosis based on physical examination alone has limited predictive power.[74,75] Chest radiography is easily obtainable and has been used as a standard for diagnosing pneumonia in the ED. Despite being commonly used, chest radiography lacks sensitivity for diagnosis and specificity in differentiating typical bacterial, atypical bacterial, and viral pneumonia. Variability among guidelines regarding the necessity for chest radiography exists, therefore chest radiography is not mandatory for evaluation but should be considered in febrile children with respiratory distress and hypoxemia in whom pneumonia or other respiratory process is suspected. Children who are dehydrated may not have an infiltrate on initial radiography.[76] Ultrasonography has emerged as another valuable tool in the evaluation of pneumonia. In addition to the obvious advantages of point of care accessibility, rapid performance, and avoidance of radiation, recent studies suggest that ultrasonography has higher sensitivity than chest radiography.[77,78] and high specificity.[79] In addition, ultrasonography compared favorably with CT in the diagnosis of pneumonia and its complications.[78] ED physicians should be aware of the evolving role of ultrasonography in the evaluation of children with respiratory distress.[80]

Management

Treatment of children with CAP depends on the severity of illness and the age of the child. One must also take into account local antibiotic resistance patterns. If aspiration is suspected, anaerobic coverage should be added. Oral antibiotics should be considered when bioavailability of the antibiotic is equivalent and the patient is tolerating treatment by mouth. In patients with mild CAP, short-course treatment regimens have been shown to have equal efficacy compared with traditional treatment durations.[81,82] Supportive care includes supplemental oxygen to maintain oxygen saturations greater than 92%. Intravenous hydration may be required for patients with poor oral intake, dehydration, and increased insensible losses. Bronchodilators may be given as indicated based on concerns for reactive airway disease or history of asthma. NPPV support or intubation may be indicated in patients with respiratory failure, although this is rare in the pediatric population. The disposition of the patient depends on age, overall appearance, comorbidity, and severity of illness. For patients who are appear well and are deemed appropriate for outpatient management, follow-up in 24 to 48 hours is recommended (**Tables 3** and **4**).

Admission should be considered in children with underlying cardiac or pulmonary disease, or children who are immunocompromised. Children with a comorbid condition and preceding influenza infection are more likely to require hospitalization than otherwise healthy children.[83,84]

Table 3
Management of children with community-acquired pneumonia

Age	Outpatient	Inpatient
Neonate	Admit patient	Ampicillin plus cefotaxime OR Ampicillin plus gentamycin If HSV likely, add acyclovir

1–3 mo	Amoxicillin
	Clarithromycin[a]
		Cefotaxime
		Cefuroxime
		If MRSA suspected add 1
		   Vancomycin
		   Clindamycin

3 mo–5 y	Amoxicillin
	If atypical likely
	   Azithromycin
	   Clarithromycin
	Alternatives
	Amoxicillin-clavulanic acid
	Cefuroxime
		Ceftriaxone
		Cefotaxime
		Cefuroxime
		If *S pneumoniae* likely add
		   Ampicillin
		If severely ill add 1
		   Vancomycin
		   Clindamycin
		If atypical suspected add
		   Macrolide IV or po[a]

5–18 y	Azithromycin
	If *S pneumoniae* likely
	   Amoxicillin
	Alternatives
	Doxycycline[b]
	Amoxicillin-clavulanic acid
	Cefuroxime
	Levofloxacin[c]
	Moxifloxacin[c]
		Ceftriaxone
		Cefuroxime
		If *S pneumoniae* likely add
		   Ampicillin
		If severely ill add 1
		   Vancomycin
		   Clindamycin
		If atypical suspected add
		   Macrolide IV or po

Constructed from the 2011 IDSA Pneumonia guideline endorsed by AAP.[73]

Abbreviations: HSV, herpes simplex virus; IV, intravenous; MRSA, methicillin-resistant *S aureus*; po, by mouth.

[a] Not approved by the US FDA in this age group. Safety and effectiveness not established for age less than 6 months.

[b] Avoid age less than 8 years because of effects on dentition.

[c] Use only if growth plates closed.

Pertussis

Epidemiology

Pertussis is an acute respiratory infection caused by *Bordatella pertussis.* After the advent of the pertussis vaccine, pertussis infections reached an all-time low; however, in the last decade there has been a relative increase in documented cases of pertussis as well as infant mortality caused by pertussis.[85–89]

Clinical Presentation

There are 3 phases of pertussis that are clinically relevant. The catarrhal phase occurs first and is characterized by cough, conjunctivitis, and coryza. It may last for 1 to 2 weeks. The catarrhal phase is followed by the paroxysmal phase, which lasts for 2 to 4 weeks. During this phase the cough worsens and becomes spasmodic in nature. There is a characteristic "whoop" caused by sudden inflow of air with inspiration between paroxysms of cough. The characteristic "whoop" may not be present in infants;

Table 4
Admission and outpatient management

Admission	Age <1 mo
	Oxygen requirement (room air oxygen <92%)
	Respiratory distress
	Toxic appearing
	Signs of sepsis
	Failure of outpatient therapy
	Complicated pneumonia on radiography[a]
	Unreliable caregiver or follow-up
Outpatient management	Well-appearing
	Uncomplicated pneumonia
	Adequate oxygenation
	Well hydrated/tolerating po
	Reliable caregiver and follow-up

Constructed from the 2011 IDSA Pneumonia guideline endorsed by AAP.[73]
[a] Effusion, empyema, pneumatocele, necrosis, lung abscess.

a staccato cough and apneic episodes have been described as characteristic in infants. The convalescent phase follows the paroxysmal phase and this is characterized by a chronic cough that may last several weeks.

Evaluation

Whereas culture of the gram-negative *B pertussis* bacteria is considered the gold standard, polymerase chain reaction testing of nasopharyngeal specimens is widely available and the most accessible means of testing and diagnosis. Leukocytosis with lymphocytic predominance is commonly found but may be absent in children less than 6 months of age. Chest radiographs are typically normal but may reveal a ragged right heart border. The presence of leukocytosis with lymphocytic predominance coupled with pulmonary infiltrates on chest radiography denotes a poor prognosis in infants.[86,87]

Box 9
Criteria for admission in patients with pertussis

- Intractable nausea and vomiting
- Dehydration
- Failure to thrive
- Apneic spells
- Seizures
- Encephalopathy
- Hypoxemia

Consider admission

- Infants younger than 3 months
- Premature infants
- Underlying pulmonary disease
- Underlying cardiac disease
- Underlying neuromuscular disease

Management

Once the patient has entered the paroxysmal phase, treatment is of minimal benefit to the patient and supportive in nature. Treatment is aimed at decreased dissemination of the disease. Macrolide therapy initiated within 3 to 4 weeks may decrease dissemination of the disease. For patients allergic to macrolides, trimethoprim-sulbactam is recommended. Patients with pertussis should be placed in isolation and prophylaxis is recommended for contacts regardless of vaccination status. In addition, maximal nutrition, hydration, and supplemental oxygen should be provided as needed. Infants should be closely monitored for apnea, cyanosis, or hypoxia. The use of corticosteroids and albuterol is not supported by controlled prospective data. Pneumonia is the most common complication of pertussis occurring in up to 20% of cases. Concomitant pneumonia is attributed to 90% of deaths from pertussis.[86] Close follow-up for repeat evaluation of hydration and nutrition status and evaluation for complications is crucial (**Box 9**).

SUMMARY

Pediatric respiratory illnesses are a significant cause of morbidity and mortality. Children with respiratory complaints commonly present to the ED and it is imperative that physicians are able to promptly recognize and treat these disease processes.

REFERENCES

1. Reilly JS, Cook SP, Stool D, et al. Prevention and management of aerodigestive foreign body injuries in childhood. Pediatr Clin North Am 1996;43:1403–11.
2. White DR, Zdanski CJ, Drake AF. Comparison of pediatric airway foreign bodies over fifty years. South Med J 2004;97:434–6.
3. Tan HK, Brown K, McGill T, et al. Airway foreign bodies (FB): a 10-year review. Int J Pediatr Otorhinolaryngol 2000;56(2):91–9.
4. Hsu W, Sheen TS, Lin CD, et al. Clinical experiences of removing foreign bodies in the airway and esophagus with a rigid endoscope: a series of 3217 cases from 1970 to 1996. Otolaryngol Head Neck Surg 2000;122(3):450–4.
5. Even L, Heno N, Talmon Y, et al. Diagnostic evaluation of foreign body aspiration in children: a prospective study. J Pediatr Surg 2005;40:1122–7.
6. Kim IG, Brummitt WM, Humphry A. Foreign body in the airway: a review of 202 cases. Laryngoscope 1973;83(3):347–54.
7. Bloom DC. Plastic laryngeal foreign bodies in children: a diagnostic challenge. Int J Pediatr Otorhinolaryngol 2005;69(5):657–62.
8. Brown JC, Chapman T, Klein EJ, et al. The utility of adding expiratory or decubitus chest radiographs to the radiographic evaluation of suspected pediatric airway foreign bodies. Ann Emerg Med 2013;61(1):19–26.
9. Adaletli I, Kurugoglu S, Ulus S, et al. Utilization of low-dose multidetector CT and virtual bronchoscopy in children with suspected foreign body aspiration. Pediatr Radiol 2007;37:33–40.
10. Zerella JT, Dimler M, McGill LC, et al. Foreign body aspiration in children: value of radiography and complications of bronchoscopy. J Pediatr Surg 1998;33(11):1651–4.
11. Righini CA, Morel N, Karkas A, et al. What is the diagnostic value of flexible bronchoscopy in the initial investigation of children with suspected foreign body aspiration? Int J Pediatr Otorhinolaryngol 2007;71:1383–90.

12. Martinot A, Closset M, Marquette CH, et al. Indications for flexible versus rigid bronchoscopy in children with suspected foreign-body aspiration. Am J Respir Crit Care Med 1997;155:1676–9.
13. Epidemiology and Statistics Unit. Trends in asthma morbidity and mortality. Washington, DC: American Lung Association. 2012.
14. Wu AC, Tantisira K, Li L, et al. Predictors of symptoms are different from predictors of severe exacerbations from asthma in children. Chest 2011;140(1):100–7.
15. Gorelick MH, Stevens MW, Schultz TR, et al. Performance of a novel clinical score, the Pediatric Asthma Severity Score (PASS), in the evaluation of acute asthma. Acad Emerg Med 2004;11(1):10–8.
16. Chalut DS, Ducharme FM, Davis G. The Preschool Respiratory Assessment Measure (PRAM): a responsive index of acute asthma severity. J Pediatr 2000;137(6): 762–8.
17. Ducharme FM, Chalut D, Plotnick L, et al. The pediatric respiratory assessment measure: a valid clinical score for assessing acute asthma severity from toddlers to teenagers. J Pediatr 2008;152(4):476–80.
18. Gouin S, Robidas I, Gravel J, et al. Prospective evaluation of two clinical scores for acute asthma in children 18 months to 7 years of age. Acad Emerg Med 2010; 17(6):598–603.
19. Cates CJ, Crilly JA, Rowe BH. Holding chambers (spacers) versus nebulisers for beta-agonist treatment of acute asthma. Cochrane Database Syst Rev 2006;(2):CD000052.
20. Closa RM, Ceballos JM, Gómez-Papí A, et al. Efficacy of bronchodilators administered by nebulizers versus spacer devices in infants with acute wheezing. Pediatr Pulmonol 1998;26(5):344–8.
21. Papo MC, Frank J, Thompson AE. A prospective, randomized study of continuous versus intermittent nebulized albuterol for severe status asthmaticus in children. Crit Care Med 1993;21.10:1479–86.
22. Camargo CA, Spooner CH, Rowe BH. Continuous versus intermittent beta-agonists for acute asthma. Cochrane Database Syst Rev 2003;(4):CD001115.
23. Ram F, Ram F, Wright J, et al. Comparison of the effectiveness of inhaler devices in asthma and chronic obstructive airways disease: a systematic review of the literature. Health Technol Assess 2001;5(26):1–149.
24. Bowton DL, Goldsmith WM, Haponik EF. Substitution of metered-dose inhalers for hand-held nebulizers. Success and cost savings in a large, acute-care hospital. Chest 1992;101(2):305–8.
25. Doan Q, Shefrin A, Johnson D. Cost-effectiveness of metered-dose inhalers for asthma exacerbations in the pediatric emergency department. Pediatrics 2011; 127(5):e1105–11.
26. Rodrigo GJ, Castro-Rodriguez JA. Anticholinergics in the treatment of children and adults with acute asthma: a systematic review with meta-analysis. Thorax 2005;60.9:740–6.
27. Plotnick L, Ducharme F. Combined inhaled anticholinergics and beta2-agonists for initial treatment of acute asthma in children. Cochrane Database Syst Rev 2000;(4):CD000060.
28. Rowe BH, Spooner C, Ducharme FM, et al. Early emergency department treatment of acute asthma with systemic corticosteroids. Cochrane Database Syst Rev 2001;(1):CD002178.
29. Bhogal SK, McGillivray D, Bourbeau J, et al. Early administration of systemic corticosteroids reduces hospital admission rates for children with moderate and severe asthma exacerbation. Ann Emerg Med 2012;60(1):84–91.

30. Rowe BH, Edmonds ML, Spooner CH, et al. Corticosteroid therapy for acute asthma. Respir Med 2004;98(4):275–84.
31. Fiel SB, Vincken W. Systemic corticosteroid therapy for acute asthma exacerbations. J Asthma 2006;43(5):321–31.
32. Zemek R, Plint A, Osmond MH, et al. Triage nurse initiation of corticosteroids in pediatric asthma is associated with improved emergency department efficiency. Pediatrics 2012;129(4):671–80.
33. Becker JM, Arora A, Scarfone RJ, et al. Oral versus intravenous corticosteroids in children hospitalized with asthma. J Allergy Clin Immunol 1999;103(4):586–90.
34. Kravitz J, Dominici P, Ufberg J, et al. Two days of dexamethasone versus 5 days of prednisone in the treatment of acute asthma: a randomized controlled trial. Ann Emerg Med 2011;58(2):200–4.
35. Greenberg RA, Kerby G, Roosevelt GE. A comparison of oral dexamethasone with oral prednisone in pediatric asthma exacerbations treated in the emergency department. Clin Pediatr 2008;47.8:817–23.
36. Shefrin AE, Goldman RD. Use of dexamethasone and prednisone in acute asthma exacerbations in pediatric patients. Can Fam Physician 2009;55(7):704.
37. Altamimi S, Robertson G, Jastaniah W, et al. Single-dose oral dexamethasone in the emergency management of children with exacerbations of mild to moderate asthma. Pediatr Emerg Care 2006;22(12):786–93.
38. Stevenson M, Opel DJ. The cost of corticosteroid choice in acute asthma. AAP Grand Rounds 2013;29(1):3.
39. Gordon S, Tompkins T, Dayan PS. Randomized trial of single-dose intramuscular dexamethasone compared with prednisolone for children with acute asthma. Pediatr Emerg Care 2007;23(8):521–7.
40. Gries DM, Moffitt DR, Pulos E, et al. A single dose of intramuscularly administered dexamethasone acetate is as effective as oral prednisone to treat asthma exacerbations in young children. J Pediatr 2000;136(3):298–303.
41. Schuh S, Dick PT, Stephens D, et al. High-dose inhaled fluticasone does not replace oral prednisolone in children with mild to moderate acute asthma. Pediatrics 2006;118(2):644–50.
42. Schuh S, Reisman J, Alshehri M, et al. A comparison of inhaled fluticasone and oral prednisone for children with severe acute asthma. N Engl J Med 2000; 343(10):689–94.
43. Rowe BH, Bretzlaff JA, Bourdon C, et al. Magnesium sulfate for treating exacerbations of acute asthma in the emergency department. Cochrane Database Syst Rev 2000;(2):CD001490.
44. Rivera ML, Kim TY, Stewart GM, et al. Albuterol nebulized in heliox in the initial ED treatment of pediatric asthma: a blinded, randomized controlled trial. Am J Emerg Med 2006;24(1):38–42.
45. Ho AMH, Lee A, Karmakar MK, et al. Heliox vs air-oxygen mixtures for the treatment of patients with acute asthma: a systematic overview. Chest 2003;123(3):882–90.
46. Rodrigo GJ, Pollack C, Rodrigo C, et al. Heliox for non-intubated acute asthma patients. Cochrane Database Syst Rev 2006;(4):CD002884.
47. Abd-Allah SA, Rogers MS, Terry M, et al. Helium-oxygen therapy for pediatric acute severe asthma requiring mechanical ventilation. Pediatr Crit Care Med 2003;4(3):353–7.
48. Rodrigo GJ. Advances in acute asthma. Curr Opin Pulm Med 2015;21(1):22–6.
49. El-Khatib MF, Jamaleddine G, Kanj N, et al. Effect of heliox-and air-driven nebulized bronchodilator therapy on lung function in patients with asthma. Lung 2014; 192(3):377–83.

50. Wong Judith JM, Lee JH, Turner DA, et al. A review of the use of adjunctive therapies in severe acute asthma exacerbation in critically ill children. Expert Rev Respir Med 2014;8(4):423–41.
51. Kline-Krammes S, Patel NH, Robinson S. Childhood asthma: a guide for pediatric emergency medicine providers. Emerg Med Clin North Am 2013;31(3):705–32.
52. Bellomo R, McLaughlin P, Tai E, et al. Asthma requiring mechanical ventilation. A low morbidity approach. Chest 1994;105(3):891–6.
53. Mallemat. ED ventilator management, in press.
54. Kamienski M. When sore throat gets serious: three different cases, three very different causes. Am J Nurs 2007;107(10):35–8.
55. Centers for Disease Control and Prevention (CDC). Progress toward eliminating *Haemophilus influenzae* type B disease among infants and children-United States, 1987-1997. MMWR Morb Mortal Wkly Rep 1998;47(46):993–8.
56. Adams WG, Deaver KA, Cochi SL, et al. Decline of childhood *Haemophilus influenzae* type b (Hib) disease in the Hib vaccine era. JAMA 1993;269(2):221–6.
57. Faden H. The dramatic change in the epidemiology of pediatric epiglottitis. Pediatr Emerg Care 2006;22(6):443–4.
58. Leboulanger N, Garabedian EN. Airway management in pediatric head and neck infections. Infect Disord Drug Targets 2012;12(4):256–60.
59. Subcommittee on Bronchiolitis. Clinical practice guideline: the diagnosis, management, and prevention or bronchiolitis. Pediatrics 2014;134:e1474–502.
60. Hasegawa K, Tsugawa Y, Brown DF, et al. Trends in bronchiolitis hospitalizations in the United States, 2000-2009. Pediatrics 2013;132(1):28–36.
61. Hall CB, Weinberg GA, Blumkin AK, et al. Respiratory syncytial virus-associated hospitalizations among children less than 24 months of age. Pediatrics 2013;132(2).
62. Swingler GH, Hussey GD, Zwarenstein M. Randomised controlled trial of clinical outcome after chest radiograph in ambulatory acute lower-respiratory infection in children. Lancet 1998;351(9100):404–8.
63. Schuh S, Lalani A, Allen U, et al. Evaluation of the utility of radiography in acute bronchiolitis. J Pediatr 2007;150(4):429–33.
64. Denny FW, Clyde WA Jr. Acute lower respiratory tract infections in nonhospitalized children. J Pediatr 1986;108(5 Pt 1):635–46.
65. Black SB, Shinefield HR, Ling S, et al. Effectiveness of heptavalent pneumococcal conjugate vaccine in children younger than five years of age for prevention of pneumonia. Pediatr Infect Dis J 2002;21(9):810–5.
66. McIntosh K. Community-acquired pneumonia in children. N Engl J Med 2003;346(6):429–37.
67. Michelow IC, Olsen K, Lozano J, et al. Epidemiology and clinical characteristics of community-acquired pneumonia in hospitalized children. Pediatrics 2004;113(4):701–7.
68. Tsolia MN, Psarras S, Bossios A, et al. Etiology of community-acquired pneumonia in hospitalized school-age children: evidence for high prevalence of viral infections. Clin Infect Dis 2004;39(5):681–6.
69. Juvén T, Mertsola J, Waris M, et al. Etiology of community-acquired pneumonia in 254 hospitalized children. Pediatr Infect Dis J 2000;19(4):293–8.
70. Lynch T, Platt R, Gouin S, et al. Can we predict which children with clinically suspected pneumonia will have the presence of focal infiltrates on chest radiographs? Pediatrics 2004;113(3 Pt 1):e186–9.
71. Mahabee-Gittens EM, Grupp-Phelan J, Brody AS, et al. Identifying children with pneumonia in the emergency department. Clin Pediatr (Phila) 2005;44(5):427–35.

72. Rothrock SG, Green SM, Fanelli JM, et al. Do published guidelines predict pneumonia in children presenting to an urban ED? Pediatr Emerg Care 2001;17(4): 240–3.

73. Bradley JS, Byington CL, Shah SS, et al. The management of community-acquired pneumonia in infants and children older than 3 months of age: clinical practice guidelines by the Pediatric Infectious Diseases Society and the Infectious Diseases Society of America. Clin Infect Dis 2011;53(7):e25–76.

74. Neuman MI, Scully KJ, Kim D, et al. Physician assessment of the likelihood of pneumonia in a pediatric emergency department. Pediatr Emerg Care 2010; 26(11):817–22.

75. Murphy CG, van de Pol AC, Harper MB, et al. Clinical predictors of occult pneumonia in the febrile child. Acad Emerg Med 2007;14(3):243–9.

76. Shah S, Sharieff GQ. Pediatric respiratory infections. Emerg Med Clin North Am 2007;25.4:961–79.

77. Cortellaro F, Colombo S, Coen D, et al. Lung ultrasound is an accurate diagnostic tool for the diagnosis of pneumonia in the emergency department. Emerg Med J 2012;29(1):19–23.

78. Kurian J, Levin TL, Han BK, et al. Comparison of ultrasound and CT in the evaluation of pneumonia complicated by parapneumonic effusion in children. Am J Roentgenol 2009;193(6):1648–54.

79. Shah VP, Tunik MG, Tsung JW. Prospective evaluation of point-of-care ultrasonography for the diagnosis of pneumonia in children and young adults. JAMA Pediatr 2013;167.2:119–25.

80. Respiratory emergencies, in press.

81. Haider BA, Lassi ZS, Bhutta ZA. Short-course versus long-course antibiotic therapy for non-severe community-acquired pneumonia in children aged 2 months to 50 months. Cochrane Database Syst Rev 2008;(2):CD005976.

82. Homier V, Bellevance C, Xhignesse M. Prevalence of pneumonia in children under 12 years of age who undergo abdominal radiography in the emergency department. CJEM 2007;9(5):347–51.

83. Dawood FS, Fiore A, Kamimoto L, et al. Influenza-associated pneumonia in children hospitalized with laboratory-confirmed influenza, 2003–2008. Pediatr Infect Dis J 2010;29:585–90.

84. Bender JM, Ampofo K, Gesteland P, et al. Development and validation of a risk score for predicting hospitalization in children with influenza virus infection. Pediatr Emerg Care 2009;25(6):369–75.

85. Vitek C, Pascual B, Murphy T. Pertussis deaths in the United States in the 1990s. Abstracts of the 40th Interscience Conference on antimicrobial agents and chemotherapy, September 17-20, 2000, Toronto, Ontario, Canada. American Society for Microbiology. Washington, DC.

86. Greenburg DP, von Konig CH, Heininger U. Health burden of pertussis in infants and children. Pediatr Infect Dis J 2005;24(Suppl 5):S39–43.

87. Winter K, Glaser C, Watt J, et al. Pertussis epidemic–California, 2014. MMWR Morb Mortal Wkly Rep 2014;63(48):1129–32.

88. Cherry JD. Epidemic pertussis in 2012—the resurgence of a vaccine-preventable disease. N Engl J Med 2012;367(9):785–7.

89. Berger JT, Carcillo JA, Shanley TP, et al. Critical pertussis illness in children, a multicenter prospective cohort study. Pediatr Crit Care Med 2013;14(4):356–65.

Airway Management of Respiratory Failure

Michael C. Overbeck, MD

KEYWORDS

- Airway management • Respiratory failure • Preoxygenation
- Rapid sequence intubation • Sedation • Difficult airway • Apneic oxygenation

KEY POINTS

- The decision to intubate a patient in respiratory distress is based on the physician's judgment as to whether the patient can maintain the airway, if ventilation and oxygenation are inadequate, and consideration of the expected clinical course.
- A careful evaluation of the patient's suitability to undergo the intubation process should occur before administration of sedative and neuromuscular blocking agents.
- Several distinct steps are followed in safely transitioning the awake, often unstable patient in need of an airway, to a sedated, stable patient with a secure airway.
- The key action in management of the airway is anticipation. Physicians should consider the barriers to airway control in advance, and be facile with the many techniques and technologies to rescue the airway should an unforeseen challenge arise.

 Video showing Demonstration of the reduction in anatomic deadspace with high flow nasal oxygen accompanies this article at http://www.emed. theclinics.com/

INTRODUCTION

Diseases of the respiratory system are the reason for 1 in 10 emergency department visits, second only to injury and poisoning.[1] Further, nonrespiratory diagnoses, including overdose, cerebrovascular accident, shock, trauma, altered mental status, or upper airway compromise, may result in significant airway compromise or gas exchange derangements that require advanced airway management.[2–5] Although the proportion of these patients who require active airway management is unknown, this subset requires disproportionately more resources, skill, and expertise to correct a deteriorating course.

Disclosure Statement: The author states no conflict of interest.
Department of Emergency Medicine, University of Colorado School of Medicine, Mail Stop B215, Leprino Building 12401, East 17th Avenue Room 712, Aurora, CO 80045, USA
E-mail address: michael.overbeck@ucdenver.edu

Emerg Med Clin N Am 34 (2016) 97–127
http://dx.doi.org/10.1016/j.emc.2015.08.007
0733-8627/16/$ – see front matter © 2016 Elsevier Inc. All rights reserved.
emed.theclinics.com

THE DECISION TO INTUBATE

Patients in respiratory distress may describe heaviness, tightness, or squeezing sensation in the chest, or simply dyspnea at rest. Clinical signs of respiratory distress include tachypnea, accessory muscle use, intercostal retractions, paradoxic abdominal muscle use, wheezing, diaphoresis, tachy-dysrhythmias or brady-dysrhythmias, altered mental status, and hypoxia. Progression from respiratory distress to respiratory failure can evolve over minutes, and is characterized by the patient's inability to accomplish adequate gas exchange to maintain oxygenation and carbon dioxide elimination. That notwithstanding, there are likely no precise blood gas parameters that define the moment of intervention in respiratory failure. The decision to secure the airway in respiratory distress is rooted in 3 basic clinical questions[6]:

1. Is the patient able to maintain the airway?
2. Is ventilation or oxygenation inadequate?
3. What is the anticipated clinical course?

Is the Patient Able to Maintain the Airway?

What tools does the emergency physician have to evaluate the patient's ability to protect the airway? Several options exist, although none seem to provide clear answers as to when intervention is warranted. The Glasgow Coma Scale (GCS) is a time-honored, reproducible tool that does afford some guidance with extreme scores. The loss of the patient's gag reflex has been promoted as another indicator for the need to secure the airway. Despite the intellectual attractiveness of this notion, the presence or absence of the gag reflex has little to do with important outcomes, like aspiration pneumonia.

Since its introduction by Teasdale and Jennette in 1974,[7] the GCS has been widely used for prognostication in patients with altered mental status. It allows a quick assessment of altered patients and demonstrates good interrater reliability. Increasingly, it is widely used throughout a range of pathology to promote consistent communication across specialties, standardize observations, and suggest anticipated clinical course.[8,9] In the setting of trauma, a GCS of 8 or lower signifies coma. Eizadi-Mood et al[10] demonstrated aspiration pneumonitis was more likely in patients with low GCS (<6) in a population of poisoned patients undergoing gastric lavage. It is widely accepted that comatose patients are unable to maintain their airway and need definitive airway management.

But is a low GCS specifically reliable enough to guide the emergency physician in the decision to intubate? Rotheray and colleagues,[11] studied a Chinese population without predominance of intoxicants or trauma, and demonstrated a wide response of airway reflexes throughout a range of GCS scores, suggesting that patients with altered mental status *have significant risk of airway complications even with moderate or high GCS scores.*

In considering whether to intervene, should the emergency physician be reassured by an intact gag reflex? Maybe not. In 111 patients presenting with altered mental status, Moulton and colleagues[12] found absent gag reflexes at all GCS scores. The investigators emphasized that an absent gag reflex is a poor indicator of the need to intervene to prevent aspiration injury (ie, intubation), but should raise concern for "at-risk" airways.

In aggregate, the answer to the question, "Can this patient maintain the airway?" is not so straightforward. The emergency physician should be aware of the limitations of any single aspect of a patient's presentation. The ultimate answer to this first question will be informed by a careful evaluation of GCS, an assessment of the patient's gag reflex, and consideration of the entire clinical picture.

Is Ventilation or Oxygenation Inadequate?

The emergency physician is expected to recognize dangerous scenarios and intervene to reverse the downward spiral with strategies that often involve positive-pressure ventilation. For example, congestive heart failure worsens with pulmonary edema, anxiety, work of breathing, and hypoxia, and devolves into demand ischemia, catecholamine surge, hypertension, increased myocardial oxygen demand, and progressively poorer cardiac performance, ultimately resulting in circulatory arrest. Similarly, the dyspnea in bronchospasm (as in asthma) results in anxiety, increased work of breathing with concomitant worsening air trapping, ineffective alveolar ventilation, and hypercarbia with hypoxia, ultimately ending in fatigue and hypoventilatory cardiorespiratory arrest. In these scenarios, earlier intervention is favored while the patient can still tolerate hypoxia, acid-base disturbances, and hemodynamic instability, which often accompany the significant physiologic hurdle that is rapid sequence intubation (RSI).

What Is the Anticipated Clinical Course?

Emergency physicians may not be pressed to intubate a patient for airway protection or optimization of pulmonary function, but may consider intubation given what lies ahead. For example, a patient with altered mental status after a fall from height may have no trouble with airway protection, oxygenation, or ventilation. But this patient may not cooperate with c-spine protection, or have a need to travel away from the emergency department for long periods of time, or possibly require sedation for painful procedures. For any of these reasons, definitive airway management should strongly be considered. Similarly, specific disease entities that threaten the upper airway, such as trauma to the chest or neck (eg, expanding neck hematoma), infectious processes involving the oropharyngeal structures (eg, Ludwig angina), or late-developing airway compromise (eg, smoke inhalation), warrant contemplation of early airway intervention.

What Is the Role of Arterial Blood Gas Values in the Decision to Intubate?

Although the emergency provider may find it alluring to obtain arterial blood gas (ABG) measurements to inform the decision of whether or not to intubate, it is a temptation to be resisted. Oxygenation (S_aO_2) can often be reliably obtained with pulse oximetry (S_pO_2)[13] and even in hypoxic or shock states, oximetry remains clinically accurate.[14] Similarly, end-tidal carbon dioxide ($P_{ET}CO_2$) can be used as a noninvasive tool to evaluate arterial carbon dioxide (P_aCO_2) with good correlation.[15] Further, continuous capnography can produce waveform morphologies that can shine light on the underlying pathology (eg, bronchospasm), as well as trend impact of interventions (eg, noninvasive ventilation).[16]

If obtained, the emergency physician must be cautious regarding apparently reassuring ABG values. These values are simply a snapshot of the patient's physiologic condition, and cannot reflect dynamic improvement or deterioration like other bedside data. For example, poor air movement, fatigue, and worsening hypoxia mandate an escalation of efforts despite recent reassuring ABG values. Similarly, improved respiratory mechanics, less anxiety, and stabilizing S_pO_2 values indicate the success of interventions regardless of ABG values. In conclusion, despite the appeal of ABG values, the patient is better served by considering the entirety of the clinical picture in the decision to proceed with intubation.

IMPORTANCE OF FIRST-PASS SUCCESS

After the decision to intubate is made, the priority in adults is to optimize the chances to place a cuffed endotracheal tube through the vocal cords on the first attempt. That is, focus on first-pass success.

That first-pass success is associated with fewer adverse events is axiomatic. Adverse events in the peri-intubation period are defined in **Table 1**. An overall adverse event rate of 11% to 15% is reported,[3,17,18] meaning that the emergency physician should expect complications in the peri-intubation period once in every 8 patients. Sakles and colleagues[19] noted that the adverse event rate triples when more than one attempt is needed (1 attempt: 14.2% vs >1 attempt: 53.1%). A similar relationship was noted by Hasegawa and colleagues.[18] This should inform the mindset as preparations are made to intubate the emergency patient.

To ensure first-pass success, a careful evaluation must be undertaken to establish the patient's suitability for RSI. In some cases, RSI may not be the most appropriate technique to secure the airway. For example, if the physician anticipates a difficult airway and has both time and a cooperative patient, awake intubation may be pursued. On the other hand, in case of respiratory arrest, the patient may not need or tolerate RSI, and a crash airway is undertaken. But there is a broad expanse of patients between those extremes that require intervention to transition rapidly and

Table 1	
Definitions of adverse events during intubation	
Adverse Event	**Definition**
Oxygen desaturation[a]	Decrease in oxygen saturation $\geq$10% or <90%
Esophageal intubation	Improper placement of ETT in esophagus, reintubation required
Mainstem intubation	Radiographic identification of the tip of the ETT in a mainstem bronchus
Hypotension	Decrease in systolic blood pressure <90 mm Hg, unexplained by ongoing disease process or trauma
Aspiration	Presence of vomit at the glottis inlet visualized during intubation in a previously clear airway
Cardiac arrest	Pulseless dysrhythmia occurring during intubation
Cuff leak	Air leak around a cuffed ETT, controlled reintubation may be required
Accidental extubation	Accidental removal of endotracheal tube, immediate reintubation required
Laryngospasm	Adduction of the vocal cords preventing passage of the ETT through the glottis inlet
Dental trauma	Fracture or avulsion of a tooth during laryngoscopy
Dysrhythmia[b]	Bradycardia or any ventricular dysrhythmia
Pneumothorax	Radiographic identification of air in the pleural space, unexplained by ongoing disease process or trauma

In descending order of occurrence, based on frequency reported in Walls et al.[3]

Abbreviation: ETT, endotracheal tube.

[a] Various investigators define desaturation differently, and was not originally reported in Walls et al.[18,19,47]

[b] Tachycardia is not considered an adverse event.

Adapted from Sakles JC, Chiu S, Mosier J, et al. The importance of first pass success when performing orotracheal intubation in the emergency department. Acad Emerg Med 2013;20:73; with permission.

safely to a controlled airway. It is this patient population that benefits from an expeditious and competent march through the process culminating in a safely intubated patient. Careful preintubation evaluation and a well-conceived plan for securing the airway are the key elements in the management of patients who require intubation.

What Can Be Done to Improve Success When Securing the Airway?

Anticipation of the any difficulty ahead is the first priority. The typical patient requiring emergent airway intervention is physiologically marginalized. Once the physician administers sedative and paralytic agents, the risks to the patient increase. As protective airway reflexes are taken away, can the patient be readily intubated? When the patient's respiratory drive is suppressed, can the patient be ventilated using bag-mask ventilation (BMV)? If the patient cannot be intubated, can an extraglottic device (EGD) be placed to provide airway protection and oxygenation temporarily? If the patient cannot be intubated and cannot be oxygenated (ie, a "CICO" situation), can the physician provide a surgical airway to rescue the patient? It is wise then to evaluate the patient in light of these questions so as to anticipate difficulties before they arise?

Evaluation of Airway Difficulty

Some may consider evaluating the patient and simply assigning a Mallampati score for quick airway assessment before RSI, but this is likely not sufficient. An association between an increased Mallampati score and airway obstruction, limited mobility, or difficult intubation has not been established.[20] A systematic review of published literature found the sensitivity and specificity of the isolated Mallampati score to be inadequate for reliably predicting a difficult airway.[21]

The "LEMON" mnemonic emphasizes a systematic evaluation of patient characteristics that improve the physician's ability to predict difficult laryngoscopy and intubate with success. Elements of the prediction tool are illustrated in **Fig. 1** and include *Look* at the external features to form an impression of the difficulty; *evaluate* the anatomy of the airway using the 3-3-2 rule; assign a *Mallampati* score to the view of the posterior pharynx; identify airway *obstruction*, and degree of *neck* mobility.[22,23] Identifying at least one difficult airway criterion predicts adverse events in 1 of every 4 intubations.[19] Overall, utilization of tools, like the LEMON mnemonic, may encourage a more detailed presedation evaluation of the airway and identify barriers to successful airway management before problems arise.

Evaluation of Difficulty in Ventilating with Bag-Mask Ventilation

Evaluation of the patient appropriateness for bag-mask ventilation (BMV) is the next important consideration before undertaking RSI. Frequently, BMV is the rescue strategy after a failed intubation attempt. Not only is it critical for the emergency provider to master this skill, but also to ensure any assistants are skilled in the technique as well. Several patient characteristics can impede effective BMV and should be sought as part of a routine preparation for definitive airway management.[22,24] In an observational study of nearly half a million adult patients undergoing general anesthesia, Kheterpal and colleagues[25] demonstrated 13 patient characteristics that predict difficulty in BMV ventilation and direct laryngoscopy. "MOANS" is a simplified mnemonic that incorporates many predictive patient characteristics.[26] The MOANS tool has been promoted to help identify patients likely to be difficult ventilate via BMV techniques (**Table 2**).

L   Look externally
Look at the patient externally for characteristics that are known to cause difficult laryngoscopy, intubation or ventilation.

E   Evaluate the 3-3-2 rule
In order to allow alignment of the pharyngeal, laryngeal and oral axes and therefore simple intubation, the following relationships should be observed. The distance between the patient's incisor teeth should be at least 3 finger breadths (3), the distance between the hyoid bone and the chin should be at least 3 finger breadths (3), and the distance between the thyroid notch and the floor of the mouth should be at least 2 finger breadths (2).

1 = Inter-incisor distance in fingers.
2 = Hyoid mental distance in fingers.
3 = Thyroid to floor of mouth in
    fingers.

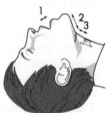

M   Mallampati
The hypopharynx should be visualized adequately. This has been done traditionally by assessing the Mallampati classification. The patient is sat upright, told to open the mouth fully and protrude the tongue as far as possible. The examiner then looks into the mouth with a light torch to assess the degree of hypopharynx visible. In the case of a supine patient, Mallampati score can be estimated by getting the patient to open the mouth fully and protrude the tongue and a laryngoscopy light can be shone into the hypopharynx from above.

| Class I: soft palate, uvula, fauces, pillars visible | Class II: soft palate, uvula, fauces visible | Class III: soft palate, base of uvula visible | Class IV: hard palate only visible |

O   Obstruction?
Any condition that can cause obstruction of the airway will make laryngoscopy and ventilation difficult. Such conditions are epiglottis, peritonsillar abscesses and trauma.

N   Neck mobility
This is a vital requirement for successful intubation. It can be assessed easily by getting the patient to place their chin down onto their chest and then to extend their neck so they are looking towards the ceiling. Patients in hard collar neck immobilization obviously have no neck movement are therefore harder to intubate.

Fig. 1. LEMON mnemonic for airway assessment. (*From* Reed MJ, Dunn MJ, McKeown DW. Can an airway assessment score predict difficulty at intubation in the emergency department? Emerg Med J 22(2):100; with permission.)

Technique of Bag-Mask Ventilation

Delivering slow, deliberate breaths to minimize insufflation of the stomach cannot be overemphasized.[27,28] Slow flow rates minimize gastric insufflation, reducing risk of vomiting. Often, in an effort to maximize ventilation, the well-intentioned assistant delivers BMV with rapid, staccatolike action. Given that the correct approach in adults emphasizes a slow positive-pressure breath delivered over 2 seconds, a single respiratory cycle can last 5 seconds or more, making the maximum respiratory rate 12 to 15 breaths per minute.

Table 2	
The MOANS mnemonic to evaluate ease of BMV	
MOANS Element	**Description**
Mask seal/Mallampati	Higher Mallampati (>2) should raise suspicion of difficulty in BMV[25] Facial hair can jeopardize the mask seal and can be overcome by applying water-soluble gel to the patient's beard.
Obesity	Defined as BMI >30 kg/m^2 and correlates with difficulty in BMV.[25,129]
Age[a]	With advanced age (>46 y old), the inferior pharyngeal sphincter muscles weaken and allow air to pass into the stomach during aggressive BMV attempts.[25,130]
No teeth	Adequate seal is difficult when the patient is edentulous. Dentures should remain in place to support the facial tissues and maintain the oropharyngeal geometry.
Snoring	Laxity and redundancy of upper airway tissues leads to snoring and can hamper attempts at BMV.[25] Elicit the history from patient or family before induction.

The MOANS mnemonic is described by Walls and Murphy[26] and incorporates many of the elements described by Kheterpal et al.[24]

Abbreviations: BMI, body mass index; BMV, bag mask ventilation.

[a] Walls et al report the age cutoff to be >49.[26]

Improvement in the effectiveness ventilation while bagging is typically accomplished through better positioning. Aligning the oral tracheal axis to effect a "sniffing position" is often achieved with a slight chin lift or a pad behind the shoulders. Consideration should be given to placement of an oral or nasopharyngeal airway to keep the posterior pharynx patent. The jaw thrust maneuver is a well-recognized technique to provide airway patency when a second person is trained in the technique.[29]

Evaluation of Suitability for Extraglottic Device

The spirit of anticipating airway management difficulties has generated a mnemonic for evaluating the suitability of extraglottic devices (EGDs) as alternative techniques for establishing an airway. Briefly "RODS" represents 4 factors that may influence ease of EGD use: *Restricted* mouth opening, preventing introduction of the EGD; *Obstruction* or *Obesity* may lead to inability to properly seat the device for an adequate seal (especially a laryngeal mask airway); *Disrupted* or *Distorted* airway, may prevent adequate seal, as in cases of epiglottitis, hematoma, or malignancy; and *Stiff*, refers to anatomy requiring inspiratory pressures that may exceed the seal pressure. It is important to remember that the RODS screening aid is based on expert opinion and the presence of one or more of the criteria would not necessarily prevent the use of an EGD.[26]

Evaluation of Difficulty in Performing Cricothyrotomy

Surgical cricothyrotomy is rare, with a frequency of 2 in 1000 airways requiring it as an initial method of airway management,[3] rising to 6 in 1000 airways when performed as a rescue alternative to RSI in civilian[30] and military populations.[31] This infrequent exposure to cricothyrotomy as a definitive technique can lead to unfamiliarity and indecision. Although this may be understandable given the rarity of task performance and prevalence of improved rescue airway adjuncts (eg, EGDs), hesitation and deliberation can be fatal.[32] For these reasons, emergency physicians must give some advance thought to surgical airway management before a patient deteriorates to the point of requiring one.

Experts have devised a systematic way to evaluate for anticipated difficulty in establishing a surgical airway. Consideration should be given to any recent *Surgery*, whereby the anatomy is distorted; presence of a *Mass*, such as a hematoma that may conceal landmarks; impaired *Access*, which may result from obesity, restricted movement, or external fixation; changes from previous *Radiation* may similarly distort landmarks; and airway *Tumors* may present challenges from identification of landmarks, to passage of the tube, to bleeding complications. Thus, the "SMART" mnemonic will remind practitioners of patient attributes that can complicate cricothyrotomy, and should be considered in advance of the need to act.[26]

THE PROCESS OF RAPID SEQUENCE INTUBATION

After assessment of the patient's need for an airway and evaluation of expected difficulties, the technique of RSI is most often used to provide ideal intubating conditions in most patients. In preparation for RSI, 7 distinct steps are recognized, from preparation through intubation and on to postintubation care, known as the "Seven Ps of RSI" **(Table 3)**.[6]

Preparation

After the assessment of the patient's airway and suitability for RSI, prepare the patient, the equipment, and the team. Ensure the patient is monitored with pulse oximetry, 3-lead electrocardiogram rhythm, and blood pressure by using a noninvasive cuff cycling frequently. $P_{ET}CO_2$ should be monitored and should be readily available after the endotracheal tube (ETT) is placed. Intravenous access should be reliable with 2 peripheral intravenous (IV) lines. In all but a few select cases (congestive heart failure), a fluid bolus will support the patient through the hemodynamic changes associated with intubation.[33]

Equipment should be reviewed for availability and function. Video laryngoscopy picture and power source should be verified. Direct laryngoscope handles with an assortment of blade sizes and shapes (eg, Mac and Miller) should be *checked for function.*

Table 3
The 7 P's of rapid-sequence intubation

Time Course	Step	Details
−10 min	Preparation	Assemble team, equipment, medications, monitors
−8 min	Preoxygenation	Maximize oxygen saturation and stores to maximize apnea time
−3 min	Pretreatment	Administer medications to provide smooth transition through RSI
Time = 0	Paralysis with induction	Sedative and paralytic medications administered in rapid sequence to provide optimal intubating conditions
+15–30 s	Positioning	Ready patient for optimal laryngoscopy
+45 s	Pass the tube with verification	Intubate the airway and prove correct ETT placement with adjuncts
+90 s	Postintubation care	Prompt titration of sedation, close monitoring for arrhythmias and hypotension, chest radiography

Abbreviations: ETT, endotracheal tube; RSI, rapid-sequence intubation.
From Walls RM. Rapid sequence intubation. In: Walls RM, Murphy MF, editors. Manual of emergency airway management. 4th edition. Philadelphia: Lippincott Williams and Wilkins; 2012. p. 228; with permission.

And ETT should be tested for balloon integrity and fitted with a stylet, with an additional smaller ETT (eg, 0.5 mm smaller internal diameter) within reach if a difficult airway is anticipated. It is prudent to have airway rescue devices close at hand (eg, laryngeal mask airway, gum-elastic bougie, and esophageal tracheal tube). The physician should also confirm suction is nearby and functioning.

Team preparation includes assembling appropriate nurses, respiratory therapists, and a pharmacist, depending on local custom. Further discussion of the physician's assessment of the need for intubation, the initial plan for RSI, including medications, postintubation sedation plan, and alternate/rescue airway management strategies, should take place. Much of this preparation can occur while the patient is undergoing a period of preoxygenation.

Evolving emphasis on checklists to standardize the approach to routine health care procedures is gaining acceptance in the care of surgical[34] and intensive care unit (ICU) patients.[35,36] Development of a preintubation checklist for trauma patients intubated in the emergency department (ED) based on accepted safety elements undertaken by Smith and colleagues,[37] demonstrated substantial risk reduction in intubation-related complications. Clinicians may find checklists increasingly useful as a tool to organize the health care team's efforts in the preparation for intubation.

Preoxygenation

In preparation for intubation, the importance of preoxygenation cannot be overstated. Through the natural course of RSI, respiratory musculature is paralyzed and airway protective mechanisms are suppressed. The time to desaturation for a patient breathing room air can be shorter than the peak effect of RSI medications (ie, <90 seconds). Therefore, the physician should endeavor to extend the period of safe apnea in every intubation. These strategies include improved positioning, preoxygenation for a period of 3 to 5 minutes, nitrogen washout, and administration of high-flow nasal oxygen simultaneous with laryngoscopy.[38,39]

How is preoxygenation accomplished?

Preoxygenation and nitrogen washout can be accomplished in most cases with high fraction of oxygen (Fio_2) applied to the airway of the awake, spontaneously breathing patient over several minutes. Nasal cannulae alone at typical flow rates (2–6 lpm) are inadequate. Widely used "non-rebreather" (NRB) masks only supply up to 70% Fio_2 when supplied with traditional oxygen flow rates (ie, 15 lpm) and self-inflating bag-mask devices can supply only 80%+ Fio_2 if a tight seal is maintained and if equipped with a 1-way valve to limit entrainment of room air.[40] In most cases, Fio_2 approaching 90% can be achieved only with typical NRB masks if the flow delivers 30 lpm, or in some situations, set to "flush."

Various approaches are reported, including "3 minutes" of breathing high Fio_2.[6,41] In a review of preoxygenation strategies, Tanoubi and colleagues[39] describe the general superiority of 3 minutes of tidal breathing $Fio_2 = 1.0$ over either 4 or 8 rapid deep breaths of $Fio_2 = 1.0$. The investigators note that if time is limited, 4 or 8 maximal breaths over 30 to 60 seconds may be advantageous in emergent situations, but this approach requires a cooperative patient and high oxygen flow rates. In more difficult cases, consider a short period of noninvasive positive pressure ventilation (NIPPV) on Fio_2 of 100% to accomplish goals of nitrogen washout and optimization of preintubation oxygen saturations.[38,42]

How long is the time to desaturation?

Benumof and colleagues[43] produced a useful model to illustrate differences in time to desaturation across various patient populations (**Fig. 2**) based on earlier theoretic

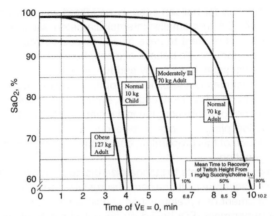

Fig. 2. Time to hemoglobin desaturation with initial FAO2 = 87%. S_aO_2 versus time of apnea for various types of patients. The mean times to recover from 1 mg/kg IV succinylcholine are depicted on the lower right-hand corner. (*From* Benumof JL, Dagg R, Benumof R. Critical hemoglobin desaturation will occur before return to an unparalyzed state following 1 mg/kg intravenous succinylcholine. Anesthesiology 1997;87(4):980; with permission.)

work on oxyhemoglobin desaturation by Farmery and Roe.[44] The message is clear: unless successful intervention to support oxygenation is accomplished, most patients will desaturate before recovery from short-acting paralytic agents occurs. Additionally, this model vividly demonstrates the heterogeneity of patient responses despite the apparently reassuring S_aO_2 at the onset of apnea. Over the past 2 decades, these concepts have been repeatedly supported by subsequent studies.

Maximizing preintubation oxygen saturation is of paramount importance. Davis and colleagues[45] demonstrated an accelerating desaturation curve for young, comatose trauma patients intubated by prehospital providers. Although a minority of patients (6%) with beginning S_pO_2 of 95% or higher desaturated during the intubation attempt, all patients with initial S_pO_2 of 93% or lower had critical desaturation.

Further complicating attempts at preoxygenation may be the predisposing pathology that initially indicated the need for intubation. Mort[46] observed that the critically ill, unstable patient does not preoxygenate adequately and desaturates rapidly. The complication of hypoxemia (simply to an S_pO_2 <90%) during emergent intubation causes a fourfold risk of cardiac arrest.[47]

Obese patients present a challenge for multiple reasons.[48] Given anatomic factors, like reduced functional residual capacity (FRC) and physiologic constraints, such as increased oxygen consumption rate (V_{O2}),[39] hypoxemia develops rapidly in the apneic period.[49] Placing obese patients in reverse Trendelenburg position of 25 to 30°[50] and applying continuous oropharyngeal oxygen[41,51] prolongs the safe apnea period in obese patients considerably.

What is the physiologic basis for apneic oxygenation?

Frumin and colleagues[52] provided an elegant discussion of the outstanding mechanism of apneic oxygenation in 1959. Assuming an apneic adult has a respiratory quotient of 1.0, and an FRC of 2000 mL filled with oxygen during the preoxygenation phase, and an average V_{O2} of 300 mL/min, all of the oxygen would be consumed in 7 minutes. Holmdahl[53] demonstrated that carbon dioxide is partitioned in the buffering systems within the tissues and blood and only about 10% of evolved CO_2 crosses the alveolar interface to be exhaled. In this example, 300 mL O_2 is absorbed from the alveolar space and only 30 mL CO_2 replaces it each minute. If alveolar volume remains constant, pressure must decrease. In aggregate, there is net reduction in alveolar pressure compared with ambient pressure at the upper airways, resulting in a driving force down the respiratory tree. Frumin and colleagues[52] observed in 8 human subjects who remained sedated, intubated, and apneic on a closed-loop circuit with $Fio_2 = 1.0$, the S_aO_2 remained $\geq 98\%$ for a duration of 18 to 55 minutes. They interpreted the gradual volume loss in the circuit's reservoir bag as "semi quantitative confirmation," of this process at work.

Such observations have led various investigators over the ensuing decades to recommend nasal cannula oxygen during apneic oxygenation at rates of 5 lpm[6,51] or 15 lpm just as induction medications are administered.[38] Aside from the mass transport of oxygen into the lungs described previously, recent work by Möller and colleagues[54] elegantly demonstrated the reduction in anatomic deadspace with high-flow nasal oxygen (15–45 lpm nasal flow). Interested readers are directed to the accompanying video 1.[55]

Pretreatment

Pretreatment agents in the critically ill patient Critically ill patients with status asthmaticus, acute coronary syndrome (ACS), or elevated intracranial pressure (ICP) can deteriorate while undergoing laryngoscopy. Repeated manipulation of the pharynx routinely causes a hyperdynamic response, which may worsen the blood pressure–heart rate product in patients with ACS, escalate ICP in the setting of impaired cerebral blood flow autoregulation, or precipitate catastrophic hemorrhage in vascular emergencies. Laryngeal stimulation can have profound respiratory effects (eg, laryngospasm, cough, and bronchospasm). Ideally, traditional agents like fentanyl or lidocaine (**Table 4**) used to mitigate injurious responses during intubation attempts would demonstrate a clear therapeutic benefit. However, unequivocal evidence

Table 4
Pretreatment medication summary

Agent	Dose	Onset	Duration of Action	Elimination	Drug Interactions	Indications
Lidocaine	1.5 mg/kg IV	45–90 s	10–20 min	Hepatic (90%); Renal excretion	Dofetilide (Dysrhythmia) Monoamine oxidase inhibitors (Hypotension) Amiodarone (Bradycardia)	Asthma Elevated ICP
Fentanyl	3 μg/kg IV	2–3 min	30–60 min	Hepatic (90%) and small intestine; Renal excretion	Cytochrome P-450 (CYP-3A4) inhibitors (macrolides, azoles, protease inhibitors) can prolong action.	To blunt hypertensive response, as in increased ICP, ACS, AAA or dissection.

Abbreviations: AAA, abdominal aortic aneurysm; ACS, acute coronary syndrome; ICP, intracranial pressure; IV, intravenous.

From Daro DA, Bush S. Pretreatment agents. In: Walls RM, Murphy MF, editors. Manual of emergency airway management. 4th edition. Philadelphia: Lippincott Williams and Wilkins; 2012. p. 235; with permission.

showing improved outcomes using pretreatment medications in the emergency patient population does not exist.[56] It had been proposed that lidocaine may have some impact on bronchospasm, but again this benefit is not supported by the literature.[57]

If pretreatment agents are deemed necessary, they should be given 3 to 5 minutes before initiation of RSI; however, rapid progression through the discrete steps leading to definitive airway management should not be delayed to incorporate pretreatment medications. Further, the real possibility of introducing unnecessary complexity or delay into the preintubation routine is a significant drawback. When weighed against the absent evidence of actual benefit, routine pretreatment with these agents during RSI in the emergent patient population cannot be uniformly recommended.

PARALYSIS WITH INDUCTION

The safe transition from an awake, spontaneously breathing patient in need of an airway to a sedated, stable patient with a secure airway is accomplished through a well-choreographed induction sequence. The pharmacologic agents facilitate this safe transition and need to rapidly meet several requirements, described in the following sections.

Provide Ideal Intubating Conditions

Rapid onset of both sedation and paralysis prevents aspiration, hypoxia, and hypercapnea. Within a narrow window, agents should facilitate excellent laryngoscopy with relaxation of laryngeal musculature, reduction in laryngospasm, and suppression of the gag reflex.

Prevent Hemodynamic Instability

Sedation with paralysis is often undertaken in unstable patients with poor cardiovascular reserve. Ideally, induction medications would have no impact on blood pressure, heart rate, cardiac contractility, and cerebral perfusion pressure.

Promote Analgesia and Amnesia

Reports of patient awareness during intubation and anesthesia do appear in the literature.[58,59] An induction regime should prevent pain, provide sedation, and facilitate amnesia to the event.

Although no single agent identified to date can meet all of the idealized characteristics, it is possible for the emergency physician to select agents that function in concert to accomplish the previously described goals. A decade ago, Sagarin and colleagues[30] reviewed frequencies of induction agents in a survey of 4513 intubations and found that etomidate was used in 69% of intubations, midazolam in 16%, fentanyl in 6%, and ketamine in 3%. It is unlikely that these proportions continue to represent physician practice today, as physician awareness of advantages of some agents (eg, ketamine or propofol) is rising while other medications fall out of favor (eg, fentanyl or midazolam). A summary of commonly used induction agents is provided in **Table 5**.

Etomidate

Etomidate is a commonly used induction agent in ED RSI. The typical dose is 0.3 mg/kg administered IV. It is generally considered to have minimal cardiovascular effects and may demonstrate neuroprotective qualities especially helpful in head-injured patients. Caution should be exercised in hypotensive patients, and the dosage should be reduced to 0.1 mg/kg IV.

Table 5
Common medications in rapid sequence intubation

	Medication	Dose	Indication	Modification in Shock States
Induction agents	Etomidate	0.3 mg/kg IV	RSI	0.1 mg/kg IV
	Propofol	0.5–1.5 mg/kg IV	May use for RSI in hemodynamically stable patients	Not indicated
	Ketamine	1–2 mg/kg IV	Hypotension Status asthmaticus	0.5 mg/kg IV
	Methohexital	1.5 mg/kg IV	Largely supplanted by etomidate, caution in hypotensive patients	0.5–0.75 mg/kg IV
	Midazolam	0.2–0.3 mg/kg IV	Considered too slow in onset for RSI	Not favored in hemodynamic instability
Paralytic agents	Succinylcholine	1.5–2.0 mg/kg	RSI in most cases Pregnancy Class C	None
	Rocuronium	1 mg/kg	RSI if succinylcholine contraindicated Pregnancy Class B	None
	Vecuronium	0.15 mg/kg	RSI if succinylcholine contraindicated Pregnancy Class C	None

Abbreviations: IV, intravenous; RSI, rapid sequence intubation.

Etomidate has been implicated in adrenal insufficiency occurring in critically ill septic patients.[60] The evidence of etomidate's role in demonstrable adrenal suppression exists, but no large studies have been completed to address clinically meaningful outcomes, such as impacts on length of stay, ventilator days, or mortality.[61] At this time, physicians deciding whether or not to use etomidate appear to have 3 choices: etomidate can be avoided entirely; etomidate can be considered for use in all but septic patients, or, given a review of the risks and benefits, etomidate can be considered for use, with the increased risk of adrenal insufficiency communicated to the inpatient team.

Propofol

Propofol is a popular induction agent for elective procedures when serial aliquots are administered to achieve the desired effect. But propofol is somewhat limited in its application in RSI of the emergency population given its tendency to cause myocardial depression and hypotension,[62] and concerns for awareness during induction.[63] Methodical titration is difficult in the setting of RSI, where the priority is rapid optimization of intubating conditions.

Ketamine

Ketamine is a dissociative anesthetic with some analgesic properties. It has centrally mediated sympathomimetic effects that can increase heart rate, support blood pressure, and improve cardiac output. Its role in induction and sedation has been reviewed recently.[64]

Reportedly, ketamine has drawbacks in head-injured patients as a cause of increased ICP. This concern is rooted in case reports[65] and small case series[66] from the early 1970s. Although no robust studies have investigated the impact of ketamine induction on ICP (the very scenario most relevant to the emergency physician), evidence is gradually accumulating to suggest that ketamine sedation has no discernible impact on cerebral perfusion pressure in traumatic brain injury (TBI). Further, with the recognition that even a single hypotensive event can increase mortality in TBI, ketamine may be a particularly attractive option for RSI in hypotensive patients.[63] Mayberg and colleagues[67] reported favorable effects of ketamine on intraoperative cerebral hemodynamics. Studies in the controlled environment of the ICU support a neuroprotective advantage of ketamine with a notable *decrease* in ICP during sedation when used in concert with other agents (propofol or benzodiazepines).[68] Thus, ketamine may have distinct advantages in head-injured populations.

Barbiturates

Methohexital is a barbiturate that has replaced the now-unavailable thiopental. It is an ultra–short-acting central nervous system depressant that promotes sedation without analgesia, and is more often used in procedural sedation rather than RSI. Dosage adjustments are warranted in unstable patients. Methohexital is known to have neuroprotective effects but lowers the seizure threshold.

Benzodiazepines

The benzodiazepine class of medications satisfies the requirements of sedation, amnesia, anxiolysis, and a degree of muscle relaxation. Midazolam is the representative agent for the purposes of RSI, with a faster onset of action than others in this class. However, significant disadvantages of midazolam as an induction agent for RSI include respiratory depression leading to apnea independent of neuromuscular blocker administration.[69] Additionally, midazolam may not reach peak effect of sedation as soon as typical neuromuscular blockers do (<2 minutes), raising the possibility of paralysis without adequate sedation. These disadvantages along with the wide range of sedation depth and dosing adjustment required in critically ill patients have rendered midazolam ill-suited as a single induction agent for RSI in the ED.[63]

PARALYTICS

Neuromuscular blockers (NMBs) are the medications that ultimately facilitate laryngoscopy, prevent laryngospasm, and enable passage of the ETT. This group of medications paralyzes skeletal muscles by 2 general mechanisms, and forms the basis of the classes of NMBs: depolarizing and nondepolarizing.

So-called depolarizing NMBs mimic the action of acetylcholine at the neuromuscular junction, resulting in an open conformation of nicotinic receptors and allowing a sodium influx to maintain a constant state of depolarization, thereby preventing muscle contraction (**Fig. 3**). Non-depolarizing NMBs competitively block acetylcholine at the nicotinic receptor, preventing a conformational change and inhibiting depolarization, and in this way block muscle contraction.

Depolarizing Neuromuscular Blockade

Succinylcholine (Sch) is the prototype depolarizing NMB used in the ED. It has rapid onset of action and provides neuromuscular blockade for 6 to 10 minutes. In adults, the typical dose is 1.5 mg/kg IV. However, some have advocated for increasing the initial dose to ensure rapid establishment of ideal intubating conditions without significant increase in recovery time.[62] Naguib and colleagues[70] demonstrated a stepwise improvement in intubating conditions with increasing doses of Sch, with the cohort

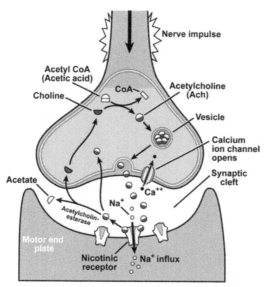

Fig. 3. Acetylcholine in the neuromuscular junction: synthesis, exocytosis, binding to the nicotinic receptor, release into synaptic space, and inactivation. (Reprinted with permission, Cleveland Clinic Center for Medical Art & Photography © 2015. All Rights Reserved.)

receiving 2 mg/kg achieving excellent intubation conditions more than 85% of the time. An appreciation for the inaccuracy in estimating a correct weight for most emergency patients[71,72] combined with a broad range of hemodynamic stability should prompt the physician to choose a higher dose of Sch for RSI in the ED.

Despite the utility and widespread popularity of Sch in RSI, there are significant side effects and specific clinical situations in which it is to be avoided (**Table 6**). Clinicians should be aware of these significant side effects, and in specific populations, choose alternative agents for achieving neuromuscular blockade.

Nondepolarizing Neuromuscular Blockade

Rocuronium is the representative nondepolarizing NMB used in RSI in the ED (see **Table 4**). It has a rapid onset of action (60 seconds) but is known to provide paralysis for up to 60 minutes. Among NMBs, it is generally considered the safest in pregnancy (Pregnancy Category B). Rocuronium is typically the first NMB chosen when Sch is contraindicated.[73]

Vecuronium is an alternative to rocuronium when the latter is not available. Vecuronium requires an initial priming dose of 0.01 mg/kg followed 3 minutes later with an RSI dose of 0.15 mg/kg. This regimen provides peak intubating conditions in 90 seconds, but in some instances results in unpredictable neuromuscular blockade onset and can last 75 minutes.

Considering the entirety of the clinical presentation is important when choosing an NMB because specific paralytic agents may demonstrate obscure disadvantages. For example, when comparing rocuronium to succinylcholine, it has been shown that patients receive sedative medications later[74,75] and in lesser amounts[76] after undergoing RSI with rocuronium, possibly leading to a paralyzed, awake patient. Emergency physicians must have an awareness of the benefits *and* risks of a selected NMB.

Table 6
Adverse effects of succinylcholine

Side Effect		Population at Risk	Management Strategy
Hyperkalemia			
Receptor upregulation	Burns	Extrajunctional receptor sensitization occurs approximately 5–7 d after as little as 8% TBSA burn.	Safe in the acute period; beyond 5 d after burn, choose nondepolarizing agent.
	Denervation	Denervating events can sensitize patients as soon as 5 d after event (eg, spinal cord injury). Progressive neuromuscular disorders, such as botulism, GBS, MS, or ALS place the patient at perpetual risk.	Any individual denervating disorder should prompt use of nondepolarizing agent.
	Crush injury	Crush injuries can result in upregulation approximately 5 d after injury.	Recent history of crush injury (<6 mo) should prompt use of nondepolarizing agent.
	Severe infection	Intra-abdominal sepsis or other serious infection may precipitate receptor upregulation over d and may put patients at risk for mo. Often seen in ICU populations.	Caution in reintubation of ICU patients with severe infection. Consider use of nondepolarizing agent.
Myopathy		Contraindicated in muscular dystrophy, as upregulation and rhabdomyolysis can be catastrophic. Black box warning against use of Sch in elective pediatric intubations.	If myopathy suspected, choose nondepolarizing agent.
Preexisting hyperkalemia		No definitive contraindication in patients at risk for hyperkalemia (eg, dialysis patients).	Consider nondepolarizing agent in hyperkalemia manifesting with ECG changes.
Prolonged neuromuscular blockade		Deficiency of pChE prolongs the half-life of Sch. Liver disease, pregnancy, burns, or exposure to cocaine, metoclopramide, or esmolol may increase apnea time 3–9 min. Congenital deficiency can prolong duration of action by several hours.	Prompt placement of definitive airway. Aggressive sedation plan to prevent "paralyzed/awake" scenario.
Malignant hyperthermia		Personal or family history of MH is an absolute contraindication to Sch. Manifestations include muscle rigidity, autonomic instability, hypoxia, hypotension, lactic acidosis, hyperkalemia, myoglobinemia and DIC. Hyperpyrexia is a late finding.	Prompt treatment with dantrolene, and consider treatment for hyperkalemia.
Trismus/masseter muscle spasm		Characterized by jaw spasm with flaccidity of extremities. Strongly consider subsequent evaluation for MH.	Jaw spasm can be overcome with an immediate dose of a nondepolarizing agent.

Abbreviations: ALS, amyotrophic lateral sclerosis; DIC, disseminated intravascular coagulopathy; ECG, electrocardiogram; GBS, Guillain-Barre syndrome; ICU, intensive care unit; MH, malignant hyperthermia; MS, multiple sclerosis; pChE, plasma cholinesterase; Sch, succinylcholine; TBSA, total body surface area.

Adapted from Caro DA, Laurin EG. Neuromuscular blocking agents. In: Walls RM, Murphy MF, editors. Manual of emergency airway management. 4th edition. Philadelphia: Lippincott Williams and Wilkins; 2012. p. 254–9; with permission.

POSITIONING

The appropriate position of the head and neck during RSI should allow direct visualization of the larynx. This often includes extension of the next to the sniffing position absent the concerns for cervical spine immobilization. If free rotation of the head is permitted by the clinical situation, the sniffing position aligns the visual axis of the mouth, pharynx, and larynx. Investigators dispute the degree of extension of the head but agree that some degree of extension facilitates improved laryngoscopy over the neutral position.[77] The advent of video laryngoscopy may diminish the importance of precise positioning, but consideration should be given to position in advance of administration of RSI medications.

Patient positioning may impact regurgitation and aspiration. Theoretically, the head-up position could decrease the chance of passive regurgitation of stomach contents, as the lower esophageal sphincter tone decreases during RSI. Opponents of this position suggest that fluids often are actively transported up the esophagus due to vomiting. In this situation, vomiting can easily overcome the vertical distance to the pharynx and subsequently proceed passively down the bronchial tree to the carina. Proponents of keeping the patient flat, or head down, assert the relative safety of this orientation in the event of vomiting, as the carina is higher than the larynx in this position, preventing aspiration.[62]

What Role Does Cricoid Pressure Have in Rapid Sequence Intubation?

Cricoid pressure, or posterior pressure on the cricoid ring to prevent regurgitation of stomach contents during anesthetic induction, was originally described by Sellick.[78] The correct performance of the procedure involves an assistant identifying the cricoid cartilage (not the thyroid cartilage) and applying posterior pressure in the supine patient to compress the esophagus between the airway and the spine. Over the past half century, the Sellick *maneuver* has been exalted as crucial,[79] and criticized as dangerous[80,81] by various investigators, but has not been shown to actually succeed in preventing aspiration during RSI in controlled trials. Patients undergoing cricoid pressure observed with endoscopy are noted at times to have significant deformation of the cricoid cartilage and airway narrowing, potentially leading to a "can't intubate, can't oxygenate" scenario.[82,83] MRI in awake subjects subjected to cricoid pressure reveals significant lateral displacement of the still-patent esophagus.[84] If the Sellick maneuver is used, physicians should be aware that difficulties with ventilation and intubation can result without an established reduction in aspiration risk.[62]

Pass the Tube with Verification

The cuffed ETT maintains a patent airway, prevents aspiration, facilitates enhanced oxygenation, and allows selection of ventilation modalities that improve acid-base status. Correct placement requires skill and improves with experience.[19,30,85]

Cormack and Lehane[86] developed a grading scale for the appearance of the glottis on direct laryngoscopy in an effort to address difficult intubations and fatal complications. Their scale remains useful today (**Fig. 4**). It is important to recognize a Cormack and Lehane (CL) grade 3 or 4 when present, as it should prompt the physician to implement an alternate plan for securing the airway. In the original work, Cormack and Lehane[86] stated the frequency of a CL grade 3 airway view is approximately 1:2000 intubations. For emergency physicians who may intubate only a small cohort of patients each year, it is important to remember that this airway characteristic is unpredictable before the intubation attempt *until* RSI medications have been given and laryngoscopy is under way, but mandates activation of a difficult airway strategy.

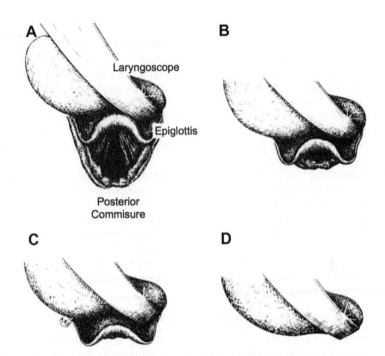

Fig. 4. CL scale evaluating the best views obtainable on direct laryngoscopy. (*A*) Most of the glottis is easily viewed, *termed* CL grade 1. (*B*) Only the posterior glottis is visible, although the arytenoids (and the cords) usually come into view with light pressure on the glottis, CL grade 2. Intubation is readily accomplished in most cases. (*C*) No part of the glottis is visible, although the epiglottis is visible, CL grade 3. Although rare, this view portends significant difficulty in intubation with direct laryngoscopy; other methods should be immediately considered. (*D*) Even the epiglottis is not seen. As it is a key landmark, slowly withdraw the laryngoscope and the epiglottis will usually fall into view. If not, this is termed a CL grade 4, and is very rare. Intubation with direct laryngoscopy is nearly impossible and other methods to secure the airway should be immediately pursued. (*From* Cormack RS, Lehane J. Difficult tracheal intubation in obstetrics. Anesthesia 1984;39:1106; with permission.)

Direct laryngoscopy (DL) enables the practitioner to pass the ETT through the cords to ensure correct placement; however, indirect methods have a role in securing the airway as well. Techniques such as fiberoptic bronchoscopy, placement of an intubating laryngeal mask airway, or using a gum-elastic bougie can all be considered indirect methods of intubation, as the ETT is not directly observed passing through the cords.[77]

Additional maneuvers can be helpful in improving laryngoscopy, including the BURP (Backward, Upward, Rightward Pressure) maneuver, in which the right hand of the intubator applies external pressure to the thyroid cartilage, and subsequently having an assistant maintain that position that allows optimal laryngoscopic view.[87] Others have redemonstrated improved laryngoscopic view with variations of this external thyroid manipulation.[88,89] It is important to remember that these manipulations are different from cricoid pressure in purpose and effect.[77]

With the advent of video laryngoscopy (VL), excellent indirect laryngoscopic views can be reliably attained in most cases, regardless of manufacturer.[90–92] VL may be especially useful in difficult glottis views (CL grade 3 or 4).[93,94] Although much of the work has been completed in elective cases (anesthesia) and controlled (ICU) settings, a growing body of work demonstrates the parallel utility of VL in the ED (**Table 7**).

Table 7
Selected studies comparing direct laryngoscopy to videolaryngoscopy

Author, Year	First-Pass Success, %		Overall Success, %		Time to Intubation, s		Cormack-Lehane Score I–II, %		VL Used	Comment
	DL	VL	DL	VL	DL	VL	DL	VL		
Abdallah et al,[131] 2011	92	86	100	90	26	38	78	86	Pen (PENTAX Europe Gmbh, Hamburg, Germany)	105 morbidly obese patients requiring intubation for elective surgery.
Brown et al,[132] 2010	NR	NR	97	NR	NR	NR	80	93[a]	Sto (Karl Storz Gmbh & Co, KG, Tuttlingen, Germany)	Evaluated glottis view of 198 emergency patients requiring intubation.
Enomoto et al,[133] 2008	NR	NR	89	100[a]	51	54	89	100[a]	Pen	203 patients maintained in manual inline stabilization to simulate difficult airway while undergoing intubation for elective surgery.
Jungbauer et al,[134] 2009	NR	NR	92	99	60	40[a]	64	90[a]	Sto	200 elective surgery patients with expected difficult airway (Mallimpati ≥III).
Malik et al,[135] 2008	88	93	NR	NR	11.6[a]	18.9	83	100[a]	Pen Gli Tru (Truphatek International Ltd, Netanya, Israel)	120 elective surgery patients maintained in manual inline stabilization to simulate difficult airway. Intubated with DL or 1 of 3 VLs.
Malik et al,[136] 2009	68	88 (Gli) 72 (Pen)	84	96 (Gli) 100 (Pen)	13	17 (Gli) 15 (Pen)	68	100 (Gli)[a] 100 (Pen)	Gli Pen	75 elective surgery patients with difficult airways randomized to intubation with DL or VL (Glidescope or Pentax AWS).
Marrel et al,[137] 2007	80	95	100	100	93	59[a]	85	100[a]	X-Li (Teleflex Medical Europe Ltd, Dublin, Ireland)	80 morbidly obese patients undergoing intubation for elective surgery.
Mosier et al,[138] 2012	68	78[a]	NR	NR	NR	NR	NR	NR	Gli (Verathon Inc, Bothell, WA)	772 consecutive emergency patients requiring intubation.
Mosier et al,[91] 2013	61	79	91	98	NR	NR	62	86	Gli or C-MAC	290 medical ICU patients intubated with either DL or VL (either Glidescope or Storz C-MAC)
Platts-Mills et al,[98] 2009	84	81	NR	NR	30	42	NR	NR	Gli	280 emergency patients
Sakles et al,[139] 2012	73	79	84	97[a]	NR	NR	83	94	C-MAC (Karl Storz Gmbh & Co, KG, Tuttlingen, Germany)	750 consecutive emergency patients. VL ultimate success superior to DL with odds ratio 12.7.
Sakles et al,[140] 2014	71	81[a]	NR	NR	NR	NR	NR	NR	Gli C-MAC	2423 emergency department intubations in patients with predicted difficult airways.

Abbreviations: C-MAC, Karl Storz C-MAC videolaryngoscopy; DL, direct laryngoscopy; Gli, Glidescope videolaryngoscopy; NR, not reported by investigators; Pen, Pentax AWS laryngoscope; Sto, Karl Storz; Tru, Truview EVO2 videolaryngoscope; VL, Videolaryngoscope; X-Li, X-lite videolaryngoscope.
[a] Reported by investigators to be significant.

Several investigators have reviewed the existing literature and it is clear that use of VL can be an effective strategy for laryngoscopy in the ED, particularly in cases of suspected cervical spine injury or anticipated difficult airway.[92,95–99]

Verification of Endotracheal Tube Placement

Visualizing the direct cannulation of the trachea with the ETT is at times difficult, and additional methods are typically used to verify positioning. Physical examination findings (auscultation of the chest and abdomen, visualization of synchronous chest movement with inspiration, or fogging in the tube) are not collectively reliable. Rising pulse oximetry readings or chest radiography cannot dependably verify tube placement. Quantitative $P_{ET}CO_2$ detection is the most accurate technology to confirm correct ETT positioning.[16,100,101] Additionally, continuous $P_{ET}CO_2$ monitoring can provide information in real time as to the correct placement of the ETT should the patient's condition deteriorate.

A growing body of literature supports the role of point-of-care ultrasound in verifying ETT placement.[102] Two overall methods have been described: direct and indirect. The direct method of verification of proper ETT placement involves tracheal imaging to demonstrate anatomic changes that occur during passage of the ETT in real time. When the probe is placed in a transverse plane at the level of the cricoid cartilage, the provider can visualize the ETT passing between the vocal cords.[103–106] Indirect confirmation of correct ETT placement has also been described[107,108] and includes documenting the absence of the esophageal shadow on transverse view at the suprasternal notch or symmetric lung slide.[106,109,110] Both findings indirectly support a correctly placed ETT. Although verification of ETT placement with ultrasound appears to be effective in skilled hands, the role of ultrasound in RSI remains to be seen.

POSTINTUBATION MANAGEMENT

Physicians who intubate patients in the ED as part of their routine duties must consider the dangers posed in the postintubation period. Even though the focus is on the events leading up to passing, securing, and verifying placement of the ETT, the physician must give careful consideration to the complexities that lie ahead in the postintubation period.

What Are the Cardiovascular Responses to Intubation?

Understanding the expected hemodynamic changes during the peri-intubation period is an important step to successfully accomplish the goal of a stabilized, intubated patient. Laryngeal manipulation, prolonged apnea with its associated hypoxia or hypercapnea, induction agents, and the evolving intrathoracic physics during the conversion from negative to positive pressure ventilation can individually or collectively precipitate a maelstrom of cardiovascular instability. Added to these variables is the unstable nature of the patient whose deteriorating condition initially prompted the decision to intubate. In aggregate, the peri-intubation period is fraught with identifiable and dynamic risks that are variably present and threaten our intention to stabilize the patient. The circumspect physician has an understanding of these risks.

Hypotension

Hypotension is common in the postintubation period[33,111,112] and has been associated with cardiac arrest.[113] Factors leading to hypotension are manifold. Myocardial depression from induction agents, loss of vascular tone in the capacitance vessels of the lower extremities after neuromuscular blocking agents, or abrupt reversal of intrathoracic pressures with the institution of positive pressure ventilation can combine to significantly impact normotension.[114] Superimposed acid-base disorders, hemorrhage, myocardial dysfunction, or distributive shock (sepsis) can heighten the risk of hypotension.

Conventional vital signs are poor predictors of patients likely to develop hypotension after intubation. However, investigators have shown *Shock Index* (SI) may serve as a marker of limited cardiovascular reserve.[115] Shock Index is defined as[116]

$$\text{Shock Index} = \frac{\text{Heart Rate}}{\text{Systolic Blood Pressure}}$$

and can clarify the hemodynamic condition of the patient. Normal range of SI is 0.5 to 0.7, and an increased SI can signal shock before overt vital sign abnormalities manifest. Heffner and colleagues[115] demonstrated an SI of 0.9 predicted postintubation hypotension with 45% sensitivity and 89% specificity and suggested an SI cutoff of 0.8 would be effective to predict occurrence of hypotension immediately after intubation.

For these reasons, continued monitoring for hypotension is paramount. As invasive continuous monitoring is often not available in patients requiring emergent intubation, rapid cycling of a noninvasive blood pressure cuff should be set on the shortest cycle time to allow close observation of evolving changes in blood pressure. If time allows, aggregating 10 or 20 minutes of blood pressure readings during the RSI preparation phase will constitute a range of normal for the patient.

If hypotension is anticipated, the physician can adjust the common approach to RSI in several ways.[117] Although not supported by large trials, administering smaller doses of induction agents in sequence may allow a satisfactory level of sedation without the abrupt sympatholytic effect of routine full-dose sedation. Volume resuscitation can be instituted in advance of RSI in all except the most obviously volume-overloaded patients. Pure vasoconstrictors like phenylephrine should be drawn up and ready, and will provide valuable pressor support during induction and the immediate postintubation period.[118] Institution of positive pressure ventilation can complicate intrathoracic physics and threaten venous return in unstable patients. It is advised to start with low positive end-expiratory pressures (eg, 5 cm H_2O or less) and lower tidal volumes (eg, 6–8 mL/kg) and titrate upward if more support is required with careful attention to hemodynamics. Ventilator management strategies of the intubated patient in the ED are covered in detail elsewhere in this issue in an article by Dr Haney Mallemat.

Prolonged, repeated, or vigorous attempts at laryngoscopy can promote increases in parasympathetic tone, leading to bradycardia and decreased cardiac output, culminating in hypotension. Esophageal sphincter laxity may result from increased parasympathetic outflow, raising the risk of emesis and aspiration. Immediate laryngoscopy before RSI agents have reached peak effect can trigger vomiting via the patient's persistent intact gag reflex.

Hypertension

Alternatively, a hyperdynamic response to laryngeal manipulation can result, worsening myocardial strain, oxygen consumption, and exacerbate congestive heart failure. Abrupt hypertension in a patient vulnerable to the consequences of hemorrhage (eg, after trauma, cerebral bleed, or vascular catastrophe) can increase morbidity. At-risk populations for a hyperdynamic response include younger patients with neurologic insult, trauma, or sepsis.[33]

Tachycardia

Despite an appropriate and well-reasoned sedation plan, patients may still manifest tachycardia and hypertension that threatens their safety and mandates some intervention. Although much work has been devoted to anticipating and overcoming these dangerous sequelae, the physician must cautiously pursue specific remedies to avoid overcorrection. If the patient is considered adequately sedated, calcium channel blockers or β-adrenergic blockers may be used for pronounced tachycardia, with emphasis on short-acting agents.[33]

What Factors Influence Sedation in the Immediate Postintubation Period?

Adequate sedation in the postintubation period is often neglected in the ED.[119,120] Consequences of inadequate or absent sedation in the intubated patient are well described in the ICU, and include anxiety, agitation, accidental extubation, loss of venous access, suboptimal ventilatory support, increased oxygen requirements, barotrauma, and increased intracranial pressure.[121]

To meet the anticipated challenges of the intubated patient, the physician must have an explicit appreciation of the attributes of a successful sedation plan.

Much of the work to date on postintubation sedation focuses on intubated ICU patients. However, the same themes of anxiolysis and pain relief parallel the goals of the emergency practitioner.[122] Enacting a sedation plan for the intubated emergency patient requires knowledge of the risks, benefits, alternatives, and indications in pursuing a particular course of action. Characteristics of specific agents are summarized in **Table 8**. Pharmacists trained in the unique environment of the ED are an invaluable resource to the physician when tailoring the individual sedation plan to the clinical situation.[75,123,124]

Lighter levels of sedation to manage agitation are associated with decreased delirium and fewer ventilator days *in ICU populations*. Validated tools (eg, the Richmond Agitation-Sedation Scale) can be used to evaluate the depth of sedation. Additionally, in the management of the ICU population, an analgesia-first approach is favored. This means that administering opiate analgesics to control pain may obviate the need for benzodiazepine use.[122]

Although subjective, pain in the critically ill patient is a source of stress that can lead to arteriolar vasoconstriction and reduced tissue oxygen tension while simultaneously precipitating a hypermetabolic state. Vital sign changes do not correlate with pain experienced by intubated patients and are unreliable in determining the need for pain medication. Using validated tools for assessing pain in the sedated patient on a frequent basis allows prompt treatment of pain and leads to improved outcomes.

Table 8
Postintubation sedative medications

Class	Drug	Onset, IV	Duration of Action	Intermittent Dosing	Infusion Rate
Opiate analgesic	Fentanyl	1–2 min	30–60 min	0.35–0.5 µg/kg q 30–60 min	0.5–1.0 µg/kg/h
	Remifentanil	1–1.5 min	3–5 min	0.5–1.5 µg/kg	0.1 µg/kg/min
	Morphine	5–10 min	3–4 h	2–4 mg IV q 1–2 h	Not typical
	Hydromorphone	5–15 min	2–3 h	0.2–0.6 mg IV q 1–2 h	Not typical
Benzodiazepine	Midazolam	2–3 min	20–30 min	0.5–1 mg IV q 10–30 min	0.025 mg/kg/h
Other	Propofol	1.5 min	2–4 min	0.25 mg/kg	25–75 µg/kg/h
	Ketamine	1 min	5–10 min	0.2–0.8 mg/kg	0.5 mg/kg/h

Abbreviations: IV, intravenous; q, every.

Parenteral opiates, when titrated effectively, are all considered equivalent and the first-line drug class for treatment of pain in most situations.[122]

MANAGEMENT OF THE FAILED AIRWAY

Failed airway is the term applied to a patient requiring a definitive airway when any of the 3 following conditions exist[26]:

Failure to maintain acceptable oxygen saturation during or after one or more failed laryngoscopic attempts oxygenation, or

Three failed attempts at orotracheal intubation by an experienced intubator, even in the setting of acceptable oxygenation, or

A single best attempt at intubation fails and a "forced to act" situation arises (combative, hypoxic, or deteriorating patient).

When the intubating physician is pressed to make important decisions quickly in a failed airway scenario, many of the sequential steps toward securing the airway that should be considered are based on expert opinion. The critical act is the advance planning, anticipation, and preparation for the difficult or failed airway *before* it occurs. Although the management of a difficult and failed airway has been reviewed from anesthesia,[125] otolaryngology,[126] and emergency medicine[22] perspectives, providers may find consensus guidelines in the anesthesia literature useful.[127] Particularly suited to the emergency physician are the emergency airway algorithms and approach advocated by Walls and colleagues.[128]

SUMMARY

Patients in respiratory distress often require airway management, including endotracheal intubation. It takes a methodical approach to transition from an unstable patient in distress with an unsecured airway, to a stable, sedated patient with a definitive airway. Through a deliberate course of advanced preparation, the emergency physician can tailor the approach to the individual clinical situation and optimize the chance of first-pass success. Sedation of the intubated patient confers physiologic benefits and should be included in the plan for airway control.

SUPPLEMENTARY DATA

Supplementary data related to this article can be found online at http://dx.doi.org/10.1016/j.emc.2015.08.007.

REFERENCES

1. National Hospital Ambulatory Medical Care Survey: 2011 emergency department summary tables. Available at: http://www.cdc.gov/nchs/data/ahcd/nhamcs_emergency/2011_ed_web_tables.pdf. Accessed May 10, 2015.
2. Sakles JC, Laurin EG, Rantapaa AA, et al. Airway management in the emergency department: a one year study of 610 tracheal intubations. Ann Emerg Med 1998;31(3):325–32.
3. Walls RM, Brown CA, Bair AE, et al. Emergency airway management: a multicenter report of 8937 emergency department intubations. J Emerg Med 2011; 41(4):347–54.
4. Navarrete-Navarro P, Rodriguez A, Reynolds N, et al. Acute respiratory distress syndrome among trauma patients: trends in ICU mortality, risk factors, complications and resource utilization. Intensive Care Med 2014;27(7):1133–40.

5. Ovassapian A, Tuncbilek M, Weitzel EK, et al. Airway management in adult patients with deep neck infections: a case series and review of the literature. Anesth Analg 2005;100(2):585–9.
6. Walls RM. Rapid sequence intubation. In: Walls RM, Murphy MF, editors. Manual of emergency airway management. Philadelphia: Lippincott Williams and Wilkins; 2012. p. 221–32.
7. Teasdale G, Jennett B. Assessment of coma and impaired consciousness. Lancet 1974;2(7872):81–4.
8. Heard K, Bebarta VS. Reliability of Glasgow coma scale for the emergency department evaluation of poisoned patients. Hum Exp Toxicol 2004;23:197–200.
9. Weir C, Bradford A, Lees K. The prognostic value of the components of the Glasgow coma scale following acute stroke. QJM 2003;96(1):67–74 (1460-2725).
10. Eizadi-Mood N, Saghaei M, Alfred S, et al. Comparative evaluation of Glasgow coma score and gag reflex in predicting aspiration pneumonitis in acute poisoning. J Crit Care 2009;24(3):470.e9–15.
11. Rotheray KR, Cheung PS, Cheung CS, et al. What is the relationship between the Glasgow coma scale and airway protective reflexes in the Chinese population? Resuscitation 2012;83(1):86–9.
12. Moulton C, Pennycook A, Makower R. Relation between Glasgow coma scale and the gag reflex. BMJ 1991;303:1240–1.
13. Nesseler N, Frenel JV, Launey Y, et al. Pulse oximetry and high-dose vasopressors: a comparison between forehead reflectance and finger transmission sensors. Intensive Care Med 2012;38(10):1718–22.
14. Wilson BJ, Cowan HJ, Lord JA, et al. The accuracy of pulse oximetry in emergency department patients with severe sepsis and septic shock: a retrospective cohort study. BMC Emerg Med 2010;10:9.
15. Santos LJ, Varon J, Pic-Aluas L, et al. Practical uses of end-tidal carbon dioxide monitoring in the emergency department. J Emerg Med 1994;12(5):633–44.
16. Nagler J, Krauss B. Capnography: a valuable tool for airway management. Emerg Med Clin North Am 2008;26(4):881–97, vii.
17. Tayal VS, Riggs RW, Marx JA, et al. Rapid-sequence intubation at an emergency medicine residency: success rate and adverse events during a two-year period. Acad Emerg Med 1999;6(1):31–7.
18. Hasegawa K, Shigemitsu K, Hagiwara Y, et al. Association between repeated intubation attempts and adverse events in emergency departments: an analysis of a multicenter prospective observational study. Ann Emerg Med 2012;60(6): 749–54.e2.
19. Sakles JC, Chiu S, Mosier J, et al. The importance of first pass success when performing orotracheal intubation in the emergency department. Acad Emerg Med 2013;20(1):71–8.
20. Reed MJ, Dunn MJ, McKeown DW. Can an airway assessment score predict difficulty at intubation in the emergency department? Emerg Med J 2005;22(2): 99–102.
21. Lee A, Fan LT, Gin T, et al. A systematic review (meta-analysis) of the accuracy of the Mallampati tests to predict the difficult airway. Anesth Analg 2006;102(6): 1867–78.
22. Vissers RJ, Gibbs MA. The high-risk airway. Emerg Med Clin North Am 2010; 28(1):203–17. ix-x.
23. Reed AP. Airway management for the uninitiated. Gastrointest Endosc Clin N Am 2008;18(4):773–82, ix.

24. Kheterpal SML, Shanks AM, Tremper KK. Prediction and outcomes of impossible mask ventilation. Anesthesiology 2009;110:891–7.
25. Kheterpal S, Healy D, Aziz MF, et al. Incidence, predictors, and outcome of difficult mask ventilation combined with difficult laryngoscopy. A report from the multicenter perioperative outcomes group. Anesthesiology 2013;119(6): 1360–9.
26. Walls RM, Murphy MF. Identification of the difficult and failed airway. In: Walls RM, Murphy MF, editors. Manual of emergency airway management. 4th edition. Philadelphia: Lippincott Williams and Wilkins; 2012. p. 8–21.
27. Ruben H, Knudsen EJ, Carugati G. Gastric inflation in relation to airway pressure. Acta Anesthesiol Scand 1961;5:107–14.
28. Aufderheide TP, Lurie KG. Death by hyperventilation: a common and life-threatening problem during cardiopulmonary resuscitation. Crit Care Med 2004;32:S345–51.
29. Albrecht E, Schoettker P. Images in clinical medicine. The jaw-thrust maneuver. N Engl J Med 2010;363(21):e32.
30. Sagarin MJ, Barton ED, Chng Y-M, et al. Airway management by US and Canadian emergency medicine residents: a multicenter analysis of more than 6,000 endotracheal intubation attempts. Ann Emerg Med 2005;46(4):328–36.
31. Schauer SG, Bellamy MA, Mabry RL, et al. A comparison of the incidence of cricothyrotomy in the deployed setting to the emergency department at a level 1 military trauma center: a descriptive analysis. Mil Med 2015;180(3 Suppl):60–3.
32. Greenland KB, Acott C, Segal R, et al. Emergency surgical airway in life-threatening acute airway emergencies–why are we so reluctant to do it? Anaesth Intensive Care 2011;39:578–84.
33. Mort TC. Complications of emergency tracheal intubation: hemodynamic alterations–part I. J Intensive Care Med 2007;22(3):157–65.
34. Weiser TG, Haynes AB, Dziekan G, et al. Effect of a 19-item surgical safety checklist during urgent operations in a global patient population. Ann Surg 2010;251(5):976–80.
35. Berenholtz SM, Lubomski LH, Weeks K, et al. Eliminating central line-associated bloodstream infections: a national patient safety imperative. Infect Control Hosp Epidemiol 2014;35(1):56–62.
36. Pronovost P, Needham D, Berenholtz S, et al. An intervention to decrease catheter-related bloodstream infections in the ICU. N Engl J Med 2006; 355(26):2725–32.
37. Smith KA, High K, Collins SP, et al. A preprocedural checklist improves the safety of emergency department intubation of trauma patients. Acad Emerg Med 2015;22(8):989–92.
38. Weingart SD, Levitan RM. Preoxygenation and prevention of desaturation during emergency airway management. Ann Emerg Med 2012;59(3):165–175 e161.
39. Tanoubi I, Drolet P, Donati F. Optimizing preoxygenation in adults. Can J Anaesth 2009;56(6):449–66.
40. Tokarczyk AJ, Greenberg SB, Vender JS. Oxygen delivery systems, inhalation therapy, and respiratory therapy. In: Hagberg CA, editor. Benumof and Hagberg's airway management. Philadelphia: Saunders; 2013. p. 301–23.
41. Baraka AS, Taha SK, Siddik-Sayyid SM, et al. Supplementation of preoxygenation in morbidly obese patients using nasopharyngeal oxygen insufflation. Anaesthesia 2007;62(8):769–73.
42. Allison M, Winters M. Non-invasive ventilation in the emergency department. Emerg Med Clin North Am, in press.

43. Benumof JL, Dagg R, Benumof R. Critical hemoglobin desaturation will occur before return to an unparalyzed state following 1 mg/kg intravenous succinylcholine. Anesthesiology 1997;87(4):979–82.
44. Farmery AD, Roe PG. A model to describe the rate of oxyhaemoglobin desaturation during apnoea. Br J Anesth 1996;76:284–91.
45. Davis DP, Hwang JQ, Dunford JV. Rate of decline in oxygen saturation at various pulse oximetry values with prehospital rapid sequence intubation. Prehosp Emerg Care 2008;12(1):46–51.
46. Mort TC. Preoxygenation in critically ill patients requiring emergency tracheal intubation. Crit Care Med 2005;33(11):2672–5.
47. Mort TC. The incidence and risk factors for cardiac arrest during emergency tracheal intubation: a justification for incorporating the ASA guidelines in the remote location. J Clin Anesth 2004;16(7):508–16.
48. Dargin J, Medzon R. Emergency department management of the airway in obese adults. Ann Emerg Med 2010;56(2):95–104.
49. Jense HG, Dubin SA, Silverstein PI, et al. Effect of obesity on safe desaturation of apnea in anesthetized humans. Anesth Analg 1991;72:89–93.
50. Dixon BJ, Dixon JB, Carden JR, et al. Preoxygenation is more effective in the 25° head-up position than in the supine position in severely obese patients. Anesthesiology 2005;102(6):1110–5.
51. Ramachandran SK, Cosnowski A, Shanks A, et al. Apneic oxygenation during prolonged laryngoscopy in obese patients: a randomized, controlled trial of nasal oxygen administration. J Clin Anesth 2010;22(3):164–8.
52. Frumin JM, Epstein RM, Cohen G. Apneic oxygenation in man. Anesthesiology 1959;20(6):789–98.
53. Holmdahl MH. Pulmonary uptake of oxygen, acid-base metabolism, and circulation during prolonged apnoea. Acta Chir Scand Suppl 1956;212:1–128.
54. Möller W, Celik G, Feng S, et al. Nasal high flow clears anatomical dead space in upper airway models. J Appl Physiol (1985) 2015;118(12):1525–32.
55. Available at: http://jap.physiology.org/content/jap/suppl/2015/04/27/japplphysiol. 00934.2014.DC1/videoS1.avi. Accessed September 26, 2015.
56. Caro DA, Bush S. Pretreatment agents. In: Walls RM, Murphy MF, editors. Manual of emergency airway management. 4th edition. Philadelphia: Lippincott Williams and Wilkins; 2012. p. 233–40.
57. Butler J, Jackson R. Best evidence topic report. Lignocaine as a pretreatment to rapid sequence intubation in patients with status asthmaticus. Emerg Med J 2005;22(10):732.
58. Kimball D, Kincaide RC, Ives C, et al. Rapid sequence intubation from the patient's perspective. West J Emerg Med 2011;12(4):365–7.
59. Sebel PS, Bowdle TA, Ghoneim MM, et al. The incidence of awareness during anesthesia: a multicenter United States study. Anesth Analg 2004;99(3):833–9.
60. Bruder EA, Ball IM, Ridi S, et al. Single induction dose of etomidate versus other induction agents for endotracheal intubation in critically ill patients [review]. Cochrane Database Syst Rev 2015;(1):CD010225.
61. Kulstad EB, Kalimullah EA, Tekwani KL, et al. Etomidate as an induction agent in septic patients: red flags or false alarms? West J Emerg Med 2010;11(2):161–72.
62. El-Orbany M, Connolly LA. Rapid sequence induction and intubation: current controversy. Anesth Analg 2010;110(5):1318–25.
63. Morris C, Perris A, Klein J, et al. Anaesthesia in haemodynamically compromised emergency patients: does ketamine represent the best choice of induction agent? Anaesthesia 2009;64(5):532–9.

64. Chang LC, Raty SR, Ortiz J, et al. The emerging use of ketamine for anesthesia and sedation in traumatic brain injuries. CNS Neurosci Ther 2013;19(6):390–5.
65. Wyte SR, Shapiro HM, Turner P, et al. Ketamine-induced intracranial hypertension. Anesthesiology 1972;36(2):174–6.
66. Shapiro HM, Wyte SR, Harris AB. Ketamine anaesthesia in patients with intracranial pathology. Br J Anaesth 1972;44(11):1200–4.
67. Mayberg TS, Lam AM, Matta BF, et al. Ketamine does not increase cerebral blood flow velocity or intracranial pressure during isoflurane/nitrous oxide anesthesia in patients undergoing craniotomy. Anesth Analg 1995;81(1):84–9.
68. Albanese J, Arnaud S, Rey M, et al. Ketamine decreases intracranial pressure and electroencephalographic activity in traumatic brain injury patients during propofol sedation. Anesthesiology 1997;87(13):1328–34.
69. Mace SE. Challenges and advances in intubation: rapid sequence intubation. Emerg Med Clin North Am 2008;26(4):1043–68.
70. Naguib M, Samarkandi AH, El-Din ME, et al. The dose of succinylcholine required for excellent endotracheal intubating conditions. Anesth Analg 2006; 102(1):151–5.
71. Anglemyer BL, Hernandez C, Brice JH, et al. The accuracy of visual estimation of body weight in the ED. Am J Emerg Med 2004;22(7):526–9.
72. Sanchez LD, Imperato J, Delapena JE, et al. Accuracy of weight estimation by ED personnel. Am J Emerg Med 2005;23(7):915–6.
73. Warr J, Thiboutot Z, Rose L, et al. Current therapeutic uses, pharmacology, and clinical considerations of neuromuscular blocking agents for critically ill adults. Ann Pharmacother 2011;45(9):1116–26.
74. Watt JM, Amini A, Traylor BR, et al. Effect of paralytic type on time to post-intubation sedative use in the emergency department. Emerg Med J 2013; 30(11):893–5.
75. Johnson EG, Meier A, Shirakbari A, et al. Impact of rocuronium and succinylcholine on sedation initiation after rapid sequence intubation. J Emerg Med 2015; 49:1–7. Available at: http://www.ncbi.nlm.nih.gov/pubmed/25797938. Accessed June 1, 2015.
76. Korinek JD, Thomas RM, Goddard LA, et al. Comparison of rocuronium and succinylcholine on postintubation sedative and analgesic dosing in the emergency department. Eur J Emerg Med 2014;21(3):206–11.
77. Berkow LC. Strategies for airway management. Best Pract Res Clin Anaesthesiol 2004;18(4):531–48.
78. Sellick BA. Cricoid pressure to control regurgitation of stomach contents during induction of anaesthesia. Lancet 1961;2(7199):404–6.
79. Ovassapian A, Salem MR. Sellick's maneuver: to do or not do. Anesth Analg 2009;109(5):1360–2.
80. Vanner RG, Pryle BJ. Regurgitation and oesophageal rupture with cricoid pressure: a cadaver study. Anaesthesia 1992;47(9):732–5.
81. Aoyama K, Takenaka I, Sata T, et al. Cricoid pressure impedes positioning and ventilation through the laryngeal mask airway. Can J Anaesth 1996;43(10): 1035–40.
82. Oh J, Lim T, Chee Y, et al. Videographic analysis of glottic view with increasing cricoid pressure force. Ann Emerg Med 2013;61(4):407–13.
83. MacG Palmer JH, Ball DR. The effect of cricoid pressure on the cricoid cartilage and vocal cords: an endoscopic study in anaesthetised patients. Anaesthesia 2000;55:260–87.

84. Smith KJ, Dobranowski J, Yip G, et al. Cricoid pressure displaces the esophagus: an observational study using magnetic resonance imaging. Anesthesiology 2003;99:60–4.

85. Sivilotti ML, Filbin MR, Murray HE, et al. Does the sedative agent facilitate emergency rapid sequence intubation? Acad Emerg Med 2003;10:612–20.

86. Cormack RS, Lehane J. Difficult tracheal intubation in obstetrics. Anaesthesia 1984;39:1105–11.

87. Knill RL. Difficult laryngoscopy made easy with a "BURP". Can J Anesth 1993; 40(3):279–82.

88. Krantz MA, Poulos JG, Chaouki K, et al. The laryngeal lift: a method to facilitate endotracheal intubation. J Clin Anesth 1993;5:297–301.

89. Benumof JL, Cooper SD. Quantitative improvement in laryngoscopic view by optimal external laryngeal manipulation. J Clin Anesth 1994;8:136–40.

90. Cooper RM, Pacey JA, Bishop MJ, et al. Early clinical experience with a new videolaryngoscope (glidescope) in 728 patients. Can J Anesth 2005;52(2):191–8.

91. Mosier JM, Whitmore SP, Bloom JW, et al. Video laryngoscopy improves intubation success and reduces esophageal intubations compared to direct laryngoscopy in the medical intensive care unit. Crit Care 2013;17:R237.

92. Niforopoulou P, Pantazopoulos I, Demestiha T, et al. Video-laryngoscopes in the adult airway management: a topical review of the literature. Acta Anaesthesiol Scand 2010;54(9):1050–61.

93. Piepho T, Fortmueller K, Heid FM, et al. Performance of the C-MAC video laryngoscope in patients after a limited glottic view using Macintosh laryngoscopy. Anaesthesia 2011;66(12):1101–5.

94. Noppens RR, Mobus S, Heid F, et al. Evaluation of the McGrath Series 5 videolaryngoscope after failed direct laryngoscopy. Anaesthesia 2010;65(7):716–20.

95. Choi HJ, Kim YM, Oh YM, et al. GlideScope video laryngoscopy versus direct laryngoscopy in the emergency department: a propensity score-matched analysis. BMJ Open 2015;5(5):e007884.

96. Griesdale DE, Liu D, McKinney J, et al. Glidescope(R) video-laryngoscopy versus direct laryngoscopy for endotracheal intubation: a systematic review and meta-analysis. Can J Anaesth 2012;59(1):41–52.

97. Healy D, Maties O, Hovord D, et al. A systematic review of the role of videolaryngoscopy in successful orotracheal intubation. BMC Anesthesiol 2012;12(32): 1–20.

98. Platts-Mills TF, Campagne D, Chinnock B, et al. A comparison of GlideScope video laryngoscopy versus direct laryngoscopy intubation in the emergency department. Acad Emerg Med 2009;16(9):866–71.

99. Mosier J, Chiu S, Patanwala AE, et al. A comparison of the GlideScope video laryngoscope to the C-MAC video laryngoscope for intubation in the emergency department. Ann Emerg Med 2013;61(4):414–420 e1.

100. Knapp S, Kofler J, Stoiser B, et al. The assessment of four different methods to verify tracheal tube placement in the critical care setting. Anesth Analg 1999;88: 766–70.

101. Neumar RW, Otto CW, Link MS, et al. Part 8: adult advanced cardiovascular life support: 2010 American Heart Association guidelines for cardiopulmonary resuscitation and emergency cardiovascular care. Circulation 2010;122(18 Suppl 3):S729–67.

102. Chou EH, Dickman E, Tsou PY, et al. Ultrasonography for confirmation of endotracheal tube placement: a systematic review and meta-analysis. Resuscitation 2015;90:97–103.

103. Kristensen MS, Teoh WH, Graumann O, et al. Ultrasonography for clinical decision-making and intervention in airway management: from the mouth to the lungs and pleurae. Insights Imaging 2014;5(2):253–79.
104. Parmar S, Mehta HK, Shah N, et al. Ultrasound: a novel tool for airway imaging. J Emerg Trauma Shock 2014;7(3):155–9.
105. Abbasi S, Farsi D, Zare MA, et al. Direct ultrasound methods: a confirmatory technique for proper endotracheal intubation in the emergency department. Eur J Emerg Med 2015;22(1):10–6.
106. Park SC, Ryu JH, Yeom SR, et al. Confirmation of endotracheal intubation by combined ultrasonographic methods in the emergency department. Emerg Med Australas 2009;21(4):293–7.
107. Gottlieb M, Bailitz JM, Christian E, et al. Accuracy of a novel ultrasound technique for confirmation of endotracheal intubation by expert and novice emergency physicians. West J Emerg Med 2014;15(7):834–9.
108. Muslu B, Sert H, Kaya A, et al. Use of sonography for rapid identification of esophageal and tracheal intubations in adult patients. J Ultrasound Med 2011;30:671–6.
109. Weaver B, Lyon M, Blaivas M. Confirmation of endotracheal tube placement after intubation using the ultrasound sliding lung sign. Acad Emerg Med 2006; 13(3):239–44.
110. Pfeiffer P, Rudolph SS, Borglum J, et al. Temporal comparison of ultrasound vs. auscultation and capnography in verification of endotracheal tube placement. Acta Anaesthesiol Scand 2011;55(10):1190–5.
111. Reich DL, Hossain S, Krol M, et al. Predictors of hypotension after induction of general anesthesia. Anesth Analg 2005;101(3):622–8.
112. Franklin C, Samuel J, Hu TC. Life-threatening hypotension associated with emergency intubation and the initiation of mechanical ventilation. Am J Emerg Med 1994;12:425–8.
113. Kim WY, Kwak MK, Ko BS, et al. Factors associated with the occurrence of cardiac arrest after emergency tracheal intubation in the emergency department. PLoS One 2014;9(11):e112779.
114. Lin CC, Chen KF, Shih CP, et al. The prognostic factors of hypotension after rapid sequence intubation. Am J Emerg Med 2008;26(8):845–51.
115. Heffner AC, Swords DS, Nussbaum ML, et al. Predictors of the complication of postintubation hypotension during emergency airway management. J Crit Care 2012;27(6):587–93.
116. Allgower M, Burri C. Shock-index. Ger Med Mon 1968;13(1):14–9.
117. Manthous CA. Avoiding circulatory complications during endotracheal intubation and initiation of positive pressure ventilation. J Emerg Med 2010;38(5): 622–31.
118. Panchal AR, Satyanarayan A, Bahadir JD, et al. Efficacy of bolus-dose phenylephrine for peri-intubation hypotension. J Emerg Med 2015. [Epub ahead of print].
119. Bonomo JB, Butler AS, Lindsell CJ, et al. Inadequate provision of postintubation anxiolysis and analgesia in the ED. Am J Emerg Med 2008;26(4): 469–72.
120. Weingart GS, Carlson JN, Callaway CW, et al. Estimates of sedation in patients undergoing endotracheal intubation in US EDs. Am J Emerg Med 2013;31(1): 222–6.
121. Gehlbach BK, Kress JP. Sedation in the intensive care unit. Curr Opin Crit Care 2002;8:290–8.

122. Barr J, Fraser GL, Puntillo K, et al. Clinical practice guidelines for the management of pain, agitation, and delirium in adult patients in the intensive care unit. Crit Care Med 2013;41(1):263–306.

123. Amini A, Faucett EA, Watt JM, et al. Effect of a pharmacist on timing of postintubation sedative and analgesic use in trauma resuscitations. Am J Health Syst Pharm 2013;70(17):1513–7.

124. Hampton JP. Rapid-sequence intubation and the role of the emergency department pharmacist. Am J Health Syst Pharm 2011;68(14):1320–30.

125. Law JA, Broemling N, Cooper RM, et al. The difficult airway with recommendations for management–Part 2–the anticipated difficult airway. Can J Anesth 2013;60:1119–38.

126. Liess BD, Scheidt TD, Templer JW. The difficult airway. Otolaryngol Clin North Am 2008;41(3):567–80, ix.

127. Apfelbaum JL, Hagberg CA, Caplan RA, et al. Practice guidelines for management of the difficult airway: an updated report by the American Society of Anesthesiologists Task Force on management of the difficult airway. Anesthesiology 2013;118(2):251–70.

128. Walls RM. The emergency airway algorithms. In: Walls RM, Murphy MF, editors. Manual of emergency airway management. 4th edition. Philadelphia: Lippincott Williams and Wilkins; 2012. p. 22–34.

129. Cattano D, Katsiampoura A, Corso RM, et al. Predictive factors for difficult mask ventilation in the obese surgical population. F1000Res 2014;3:239. Available at: http://f1000research.com/articles/3-239/v1. Accessed June 1, 2015.

130. Mittal RK. Motor function of the pharynx, esophagus, and its sphincters. Upper esophageal sphincter. San Rafael (CA): Morgan & Claypool Life Sciences; 2011.

131. Abdallah R, Galway U, You J, et al. A randomized comparison between the Pentax AWS video laryngoscope and the Macintosh laryngoscope in morbidly obese patients. Anesth Analg 2011;113(5):1082–7.

132. Brown CA 3rd, Bair AE, Pallin DJ, et al. National emergency airway registry I. Improved glottic exposure with the video Macintosh laryngoscope in adult emergency department tracheal intubations. Ann Emerg Med 2010;56(2):83–8.

133. Enomoto Y, Asai T, Arai T, et al. Pentax-AWS, a new videolaryngoscope, is more effective than the Macintosh laryngoscope for tracheal intubation in patients with restricted neck movements: a randomized comparative study. Br J Anaesth 2008;100(4):544–8.

134. Jungbauer A, Schumann M, Brunkhorst V, et al. Expected difficult tracheal intubation: a prospective comparison of direct laryngoscopy and video laryngoscopy in 200 patients. Br J Anaesth 2009;102(4):546–50.

135. Malik MA, Maharaj CH, Harte BH, et al. Comparison of Macintosh, Truview EVO2, Glidescope, and Airwayscope laryngoscope use in patients with cervical spine immobilization. Br J Anaesth 2008;101(5):723–30.

136. Malik MA, Subramaniam R, Maharaj CH, et al. Randomized controlled trial of the Pentax AWS, Glidescope, and Macintosh laryngoscopes in predicted difficult intubation. Br J Anaesth 2009;103(5):761–8.

137. Marrel J, Blanc C, Frascarolo P, et al. Videolaryngoscopy improves intubation condition in morbidly obese patients. Eur J Anaesthesiol 2007;24(12):1045–9.

138. Mosier JM, Stolz U, Chiu S, et al. Difficult airway management in the emergency department: GlideScope videolaryngoscopy compared to direct laryngoscopy. J Emerg Med 2012;42(6):629–34.

139. Sakles JC, Mosier J, Chiu S, et al. A comparison of the C-MAC video laryngo-scope to the Macintosh direct laryngoscope for intubation in the emergency department. Ann Emerg Med 2012;60(6):739–48.
140. Sakles JC, Patanwala AE, Mosier JM, et al. Comparison of video laryngoscopy to direct laryngoscopy for intubation of patients with difficult airway characteristics in the emergency department. Intern Emerg Med 2014;9(1):93–8.

Approach to Adult Patients with Acute Dyspnea

Elizabeth DeVos, MD, MPH, Lisa Jacobson, MD*

KEYWORDS

- Dyspnea • Shortness of breath • Asthma • COPD • Respiratory compensation
- Pneumonia • Pulmonary embolism • Angina

KEY POINTS

- The cause of dyspnea is often evident from a complete history and physical examination.
- Rapid determination of the cause of dyspnea saves lives.
- Shortness of breath is not always primarily a pulmonary problem.
- Understanding the pathophysiology of each disease allows clinicians to make rational decisions about testing.

INTRODUCTION

Emergency Medical Services (EMS) calls en route with a 45-year-old woman who has a history of congestive heart failure, chronic bronchitis, morbid obesity, and diabetes. She is breathing 40 times per minute, maintaining oxygen saturations of 94%. She appears mildly confused. You have 5 minutes to consider algorithms before the patient arrives. Perhaps respiratory therapy is paged to supply a ventilator or a biphasic positive airway pressure (BIPAP) machine. Maybe you prepare airway equipment or ask your nursing staff to access medication in advance, or you might use the time to expand your differential and determine what brief information regarding the patient's history and initial physical examination will help you treat her.

Acutely dyspneic patients present in various ways. Are the lungs full of fluid or pus? Did the throat swell shut or is the patient just anxious? Did the patient aspirate a foreign body or have a slow or rapid hemorrhage? Is the patient compensating for a severe metabolic acidosis or did the patient run out of beta agonists at home? This article provides helpful guidelines in the assessment and management of these diverse patients.

Disclosures: None.
Department of Emergency Medicine, University of Florida College of Medicine - Jacksonville, 655 West 8th Street, Jacksonville, FL 32209, USA
* Corresponding author.
E-mail address: Lisa.Jacobson@jax.ufl.edu

Emerg Med Clin N Am 34 (2016) 129–149
http://dx.doi.org/10.1016/j.emc.2015.08.008
0733-8627/16/$ – see front matter © 2016 Elsevier Inc. All rights reserved.

emed.theclinics.com

Respiratory distress is responsible for nearly 4 million emergency department (ED) visits each year and is one of the most common presenting complaints in the elderly.[1] When a patient presents with dyspnea, the primary task of the emergency physician is to assess for and ensure stability of the patient's airway, breathing, and circulation. In the case of dyspnea, presentations may range from minor symptoms to extremis. Rapid assessment may necessitate the use of intubation, BIPAP, nebulizations, decompression, or other therapies in the immediate period following the patient's arrival, to treat dyspnea.

PATIENT EVALUATION

The American Thoracic Society suggests that "dyspnea results from a … mismatch between central respiratory motor activity and incoming afferent information from receptors in the airways, lungs and chest wall structures."[2] This dissociation can result from increased metabolic demand, decreased compliance, increased dead-space volume, or many other disorders that are discussed later. Each patient presenting short of breath uses a different set of phrases to describe the symptoms and examination reveals a different combination of disorders. The clinician's ability to interpret these varying constellations is necessary to provide appropriate treatment to these patients, who are often in serious distress.

History

Acute dyspnea, or shortness of breath, is one of the most common chief complaints in the ED. The differential diagnosis includes many disorders that can be divided based on obstructive, parenchymal, cardiac, and compensatory features. A careful history can begin to narrow this wide differential. In addition to common symptoms, consider risk factors such as past medical and family history, trauma, travel, medications, and exposures.

Schwartzstein and Lewis[3] use the analogy of a machine to identify different causes of dyspnea based on pathophysiologic data. Dysfunctions of the respiratory system may be caused by faulty controllers, ventilatory pumps, or gas exchangers (**Table 1**). This table makes it easier to understand the causes of shortness of breath related to respiratory causes.

Cardiovascular disease manifests as dyspnea by causing disruptions of the system that pumps oxygenated blood to tissues and then transports the carbon dioxide back to the lung. Decreases in cardiac output or increases in resistance limit oxygen delivery. Similarly, decreased oxygen carrying capacity in anemia plays a role in its presentation with dyspnea.

Physical Examination

A detailed physical examination also provides important guidance (**Table 2**). Respiratory rate and oxygen saturation are obtained with vital signs. The clinician should assess the patient's work of breathing, looking for any tripoding or retractions. Crepitance in the chest may indicate subcutaneous air and pneumothorax. Lung sounds such as wheezing, rales, and rhonchi further guide the differential. Decreased sounds, hyperresonance, or egophony may also provide additional clues.

Jugular venous distension, S3 gallop, and peripheral edema indicate that a patient has fluid overload. Conjunctival pallor, capillary refill, and temperature of extremities can provide clues about blood volume and general circulation. Pulses must also be assessed.

Table 1
A systemic approach to dyspnea by assessing the components of the respiratory process

Part	Description	Manifestations	Examples
Controller	Malfunction presents as abnormal respiratory rate or depth. Often related to abnormal feedback to brain from other parts of the system	Air hunger, need to breathe	Abnormal feedback to brain from other systems. Metabolic acidosis, anxiety
Ventilatory pump	Composed of muscles, nerves that signal the controller, chest wall, and pleura that create negative thoracic pressure, airways and alveoli allowing flow from atmosphere and gas exchange	Increased work of breathing, low tidal volumes	Neuromuscular problems (eg, Guillain-Barré), decreased chest wall compliance, pneumothorax, pneumonia, bronchospasm (COPD, asthma)
Gas exchanger	Oxygen and carbon dioxide cross the pulmonary capillaries in the alveoli. Membrane destruction or interruption of the interface between the gas and capillaries by fluid or inflammatory cells limit gas exchange	Increased respiratory drive, hypoxemia, chronic hypercapnia	Emphysema, pneumonia, pulmonary edema, pleural effusion, hemothorax

Adapted from Schwartzstein RM, Lewis A. Dyspnea. In: Broaddus V, Mason RC, Ernst JD, et al, editors. Murray & Nadel's textbook of respiratory medicine. Elsevier health sciences. 6th edition. Philadelphia: Saunders/Elsevier; 2015.

Testing

Multiple tests are available to narrow the differential diagnosis of acute dyspnea. When using tests to augment clinical decision making, be sure to weigh the information they may provide with any risks involved in performing the tests (**Table 3**).

Ultrasonography provides valuable information about the origin of symptoms, and, often, diagnosis in the initial assessment of an acutely dyspneic patient. These images may be obtained during or shortly after initial assessment, potentially

Table 2
Physical examination findings and correlating diagnoses

Symptom	Differential Diagnosis
Wheeze	COPD/emphysema, asthma, allergic reaction, CHF (cardiac wheeze)
Cough	Pneumonia, asthma, COPD/emphysema
Pleuritic chest pain	Pneumonia, pulmonary embolism, pneumothorax, COPD, asthma
Orthopnea	Acute heart failure
Fever	Pneumonia, bronchitis, TB, malignancy
Hemoptysis	Pneumonia, TB, pulmonary embolism, malignancy
Edema	Acute heart failure, pulmonary embolism (unilateral)
pulmonary edema	Acute and chronic heart failure, end stage renal and liver diseases, ARDS (sepsis)
Tachypnea alone	pulmonary embolism, acidosis (including aspirin toxicity), anxiety

Abbreviations: ARDS, acute respiratory distress syndrome; CHF, congestive heart failure; COPD, chronic obstructive pulmonary disease; TB, tuberculosis.

Table 3
Diagnostic testing for dyspneic patients

Test	General Information	Pros	Cons
Chest radiograph	Often primary imaging	Low radiation, can assess consolidation, pleural fluid, hyperinflation, pneumothorax, and subcutaneous air. Heart size is apparent	Low sensitivity in acute dyspnea. In one series only 8 of 26 pneumonias diagnosed on CT met CXR criteria[37]
Ultrasonography	Multiple protocols to assess acute dyspnea	No radiation, fast, reproducible bedside test, can be done on unstable patients in department and in semirecumbent position	Requires some skill to acquire and interpret bedside images. Patient factors such as subcutaneous air, body habitus, and so forth may limit images
D-dimer	Marker of fibrinolytic activity. When measured by ELISA or second-generation latex agglutination can be used to rule out PE in selected patients	Serum test readily available	Requires risk assessment and clear clinical question. Also increased in consumptive coagulopathy, infection, malignancy, trauma, dissection, preeclampsia, and other cardiovascular disorders
Arterial blood gas	Provides additional information about ventilation ($Paco_2$) to patients with reliable pulse oximetry and bicarbonate level available on BMP	May be faster than general laboratory tests. Useful in assessing anxiety-induced hyperventilation[36]	Limited evidence for routine use in undifferentiated dyspnea
Electrocardiogram	Initial cardiac assessment for assessing dyspnea	Fast and inexpensive. Easy to compare with prior examinations. Specific for dysrhythmias or ACS limiting perfusion	May be nonspecific in findings such as right heart strain and P pulmonale
Troponin	Serum indicator of myocardial damage	Serum test readily available	Can narrow differential to cardiac causes. PE with right heart strain may have increased troponin levels; this finding predicts worse outcomes
BNP and proBNP	Useful in assessing for acute heart failure	Serum test readily available	Limited in obesity, mitral regurgitation, flash pulmonary edema, and renal insufficiency. Context is essential

(continued on next page)

Test	General Information	Pros	Cons
Table 3 *(continued)*			
Complete blood count	Provides information about oxygen carrying capacity based on hemoglobin and hematocrit. White blood cell count may indicate infection	Serum test readily available	Nonspecific
CT scan	Provides detailed imaging of cardiorespiratory system. Use is increasing, but practitioners should maintain clinical context and consider whether other modalities can answer the clinical question	Offers sensitive and specific results	Significant radiation exposure, contrast nephropathy, intravenous contrast dye reactions
Ventilation/ perfusion scan	Radiolabeled aerosol and albumin aggregates are used to study ventilation and perfusion. Read as negative or low, medium or high probability for pulmonary embolism	Low in radiation	Limited by underlying pulmonary disease and availability of isotopes

Abbreviations: ACS, acute coronary syndrome; BMP, basic metabolic panel; BNP, B-type natriuretic peptide; CT, computed tomography; CXR, chest radiograph; ELISA, enzyme-linked immunosorbent assay; proBNP, pro–B-type natriuretic peptide.

guiding therapy faster than laboratory tests or other imaging studies would be available. The Bedside Lung Ultrasonography in Emergency (BLUE) protocol offers one approach to differentiate several causes of respiratory failure (**Table 4** and **Figs. 1–9**).

Other protocols include assessments to assess for other cardiac causes of dyspnea.[4–6] Focused evaluation of global left ventricular function, diastolic function, right ventricular size, and any pericardial effusion facilitates rapid assessment for massive myocardial infarction, cardiac tamponade, and massive pulmonary embolism at the bedside. In addition, inferior vena cava measurement can be used to assess for right-sided heart failure and to estimate central venous pressure.

Computed tomography (CT) use to evaluate acute dyspnea has increased in the last decade.[7] Risks include contrast reactions and nephropathy as well as radiation-induced cancers.[8] Recent American College of Physicians recommendations advocate avoidance of CT as an initial test to evaluate patients at low risk for pulmonary embolism (PE).[9] Further, nearly one-fourth of patients undergoing CT for PE evaluation

Table 4
BLUE protocol

Ultrasonography Finding	Ultrasonography Approach	Description	Clinical Meaning	Image
Assess for artifacts: A lines	Anterior	Subpleural air causes repeated linear artifacts parallel to the pleural line (horizontal)	Air in lung: either normal or pneumothorax	**Fig. 1**
Assess for artifacts: B lines	Anterior	Seven features: hyperechoic, well-defined, hydroaeric comet-tail artifacts arising from the pleural line. They spread upwards indefinitely and obscure A lines. When lung sliding is present, they move with the lung	Represents an interface of 2 widely different transmissions of ultrasound waves: in this case, air and fluid. When 3 or more B lines are in a single interspace, they are B+ lines (or pulmonary rockets), indicating interstitial syndrome	**Fig. 2**
Assess for lung sliding	Anterior	Absence of lung sliding occurs with a disruption of the normal sliding of viscera on parietal pleura or separation of the two. In M mode, absence of lung slide is seen as the stratosphere sign (also known as bar-code sign)	Absence of lung sliding in the presence of A lines necessitates search for pneumothorax. Lung point is the ultrasonography finding in which lung slide is seen in the same view with the abolished lung slide and A lines in the same location, indicating the tip of the lung	**Fig. 3** (stratosphere sign) **Fig. 4** (normal lung) **Fig. 5** (lung point)
Assess for alveolar consolidation or pleural effusion (posterolateral alveolar and/or pleural syndrome)	Lateral subposterior	The classic anechoic, dependent pattern may be inconsistent. Other findings include (1) quad sign: pleural effusion on expiration noted between the pleural and regular, lower lung lines (viscera). (2) Shred sign: tissuelike pattern seen with alveolar consolidation, with the upper border of lung line (or pleural line when there is no effusion) with an irregular lower border. (3) Sinusoid sign: movement of the lung line toward the pleural line in inspiration	Pleural effusion: sinusoid, plus may have quad sign. Alveolar consolidation: tissuelike appearance or shred sign, absent lung line, absent sinusoidal sign	**Figs. 6 and 7** (pleural effusion) **Fig. 8** (tissuelike lung) **Fig. 9** (sinusoidal)
Deep venous thrombosis	Femoral veins	Visualization of thrombus in the lumen or lack of compressibility is positive test	Consider pulmonary embolus if positive	—

Adapted from Lichtenstein DA, Mezière GA. Relevance of lung ultrasound in the diagnosis of acute respiratory failure: the BLUE protocol. Chest 2008;134(1):117–25; *and Courtesy of* Petra Duran, MD, RDMS, University of Florida College of Medicine-Jacksonville (FL).

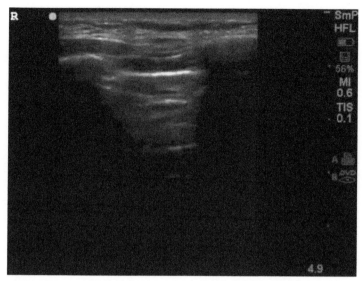

Fig. 1. A lines.

have clinically significant incidental findings. Although CT may provide vital diagnostic information, clinicians must not only consider the scan's necessity but also plan appropriate follow-up for any clinically important incidental findings.[10] Always consider whether CT is necessary or whether less risky modalities, such as chest radiograph or ultrasonography, will answer pertinent questions.

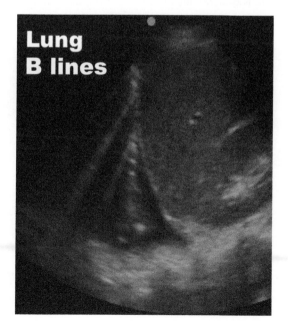

Fig. 2. B lines.

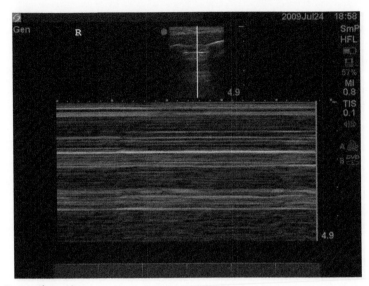

Fig. 3. Stratosphere sign.

DIFFERENTIAL DIAGNOSIS FOR ACUTELY DYSPNEIC PATIENTS
Obstructive Dyspnea

Consider the 35-year-old woman discussed earlier. Medics report tachypnea with very poor air movement during transport. As she rolls through the ambulance bay doors, you are already assessing her. Adept clinicians can spot respiratory distress from across the room. She is diaphoretic, her shoulders are held adjacent to her ears, and she is breathing extremely rapidly with minimal air movement. You decide

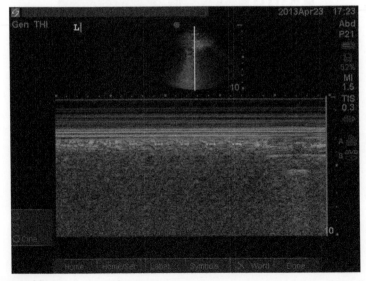

Fig. 4. Normal lung.

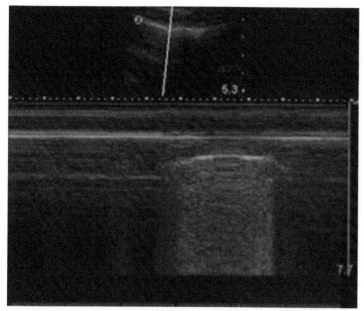

Fig. 5. Lung point.

to aggressively treat her for a severe asthma exacerbation, starting BIPAP ventilation with continuous nebulized albuterol and order adjunct therapies including intravenous steroids, intravenous magnesium, and intramuscular epinephrine. After 20 minutes at her bedside, she begins to breathe more comfortably with the BIPAP machine and repeat auscultation reveals diffuse wheezing and improved air movement.

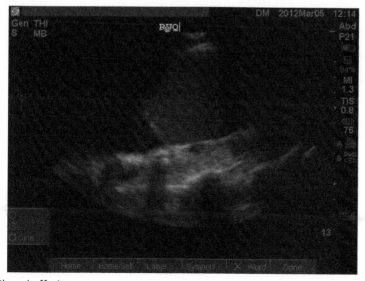

Fig. 6. Pleural effusion.

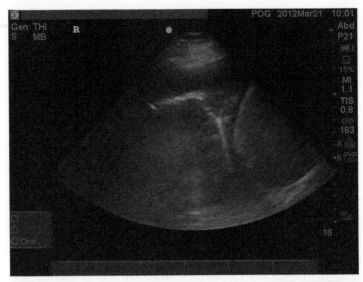

Fig. 7. Pleural effusion.

As she begins to improve, EMS returns with another patient. His breath sounds are audible to everyone in the resuscitation bay. He appears diaphoretic and panicked. Examination reveals stridor, periorbital edema, tachycardia, and hypotension. Immediate intervention for anaphylactic shock begins and, after 2 rounds of epinephrine, fluid boluses, antihistamines, and steroids, he too begins to look better.

Wheezing, or musical respiratory sounds, typically result from partial airway obstruction.[11] Because this obstruction can result from inflammation, secretions, or even a foreign body, patients with noisy or whistling breathing need close evaluation to

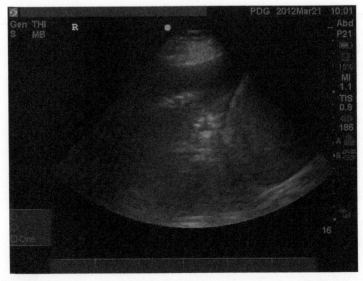

Fig. 8. Tissuelike lung.

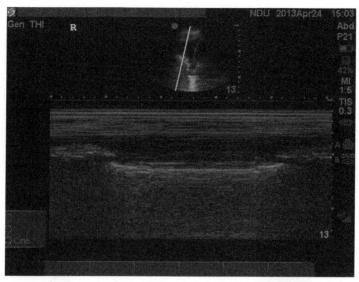

Fig. 9. Sinusoidal sign.

determine whether the noise is inspiratory or expiratory, and whether it is from the lower airways or the upper airways. Stridor from a swollen airway, foreign body, or other airway obstruction is imminently dangerous. Although patients in anaphylaxis may benefit from the nebulized beta-agonist treatment used to treat an asthma exacerbation, it is not sufficient to save their lives. As opposed to wheezing, which is a lower airway expiratory sound, stridor is an upper airway sound transmitted when there is obstruction to the inflow of air during inspiration. The obstruction may be fixed (food bolus; **Fig. 10**) or inflammatory (anaphylaxis), but in any situation must be emergently managed.

National and world organizations define asthma "by the history of respiratory symptoms such as wheeze, shortness of breath, chest tightness and cough that vary over time and in intensity, together with variable expiratory airflow limitation."[12] The reversibility of airflow obstruction is the hallmark distinguishing asthma from other obstructive respiratory disorders. In contrast, chronic obstructive pulmonary disease (COPD)/emphysema is defined as "persistent airflow limitation that is usually progressive and associated with enhanced chronic inflammatory responses in the airways and the lungs."[12] These patients also frequently wheeze, but may have a different course of acute and chronic disease. **Table 5** highlights the differences between these similar, at times overlapping, diseases.

Asthma is an obstructive disease resulting from increased airway resistance. It is a reversible but recurrent chronic inflammatory disorder that characteristically causes severe dyspnea, wheezing, and coughing.[13] There are 2 main problems in asthma: chronically inflamed airways and hyperresponsive airways. Intermittent airflow obstruction in symptomatic patients results in decreased ability to expire, leading to hyperinflation, stenting open the alveoli, and increasing the work of breathing. Early in an exacerbation, symptoms are bronchospastic secondary to smooth muscle contraction. As an episode progresses, inflammatory changes in the airways can cause increased airway resistance and lead to VQ mismatch (**Fig. 11**). The severity of an exacerbation can be assessed clinically and should dictate how aggressively a patient is treated (**Table 6**).

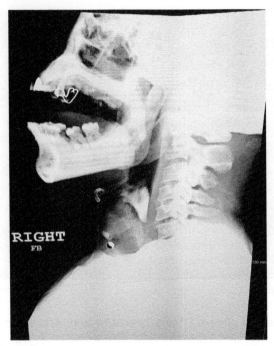

Fig. 10. Food bolus in airway.

COPD is defined by the Global Initiative for Chronic Obstructive Lung Disease (GOLD) as "persistent airflow limitation that is usually progressive and associated with an enhanced chronic inflammatory response in the airways and the lung to noxious particles or gases."[12] The pathophysiology in each patient is typically a mix of lung parenchymal destruction, as seen in emphysema, and small airway inflammation with airway obstruction, or obstructive bronchiolitis.[11] An exacerbation of COPD presents as dyspnea, cough, and increased sputum production. In the emergent

Table 5
Features suggesting asthma or COPD

Favors Asthma	Favors COPD
Onset in childhood	Onset in adulthood
Symptoms vary over time	Symptoms persist even with treatment
Symptoms worse at night	Daily symptoms, some days better than others
Symptoms may be triggered by allergens or exercise	Chronic cough and sputum unrelated to triggers
Variable airflow obstruction	Persistent airflow obstruction
Normal lung function when asymptomatic	Abnormal lung function when asymptomatic
Atopy in self or family	Smoker
No progression over time	Progression over time

Adapted from Global Initiative for Asthma. Diagnosis of diseases of chronic airflow limitation: asthma, COPD and asthma-COPD overlap syndrome (ACOS). 2015. Available at: http://www.ginasthma.org/documents/14/Asthma%2C-COPD-and-Asthma-COPD-Overlap-Syndrome-%28AC OS%29. Accessed May 1, 2015.

Pathophysiology

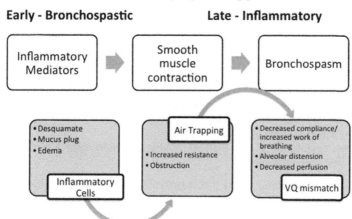

Fig. 11. Pathophysiology of symptom development in asthma.

setting, clinicians must treat the airflow limitation. As with asthma, monitoring of pulse oximetry, degree of respiratory distress, and hemodynamic stability can help clinicians anticipate the degree of severity of a particular exacerbation. More specific testing may also have a role, because radiographs and electrocardiograms may help differentiate other causes of shortness of breath from a COPD exacerbation. In addition, an increase in sputum production or the presence of purulent sputum should be treated with antibiotics, regardless of other infectious symptoms.[14]

Anaphylaxis is a sudden, potentially fatal, allergic reaction involving multiple organ systems.[15,16] The Second Symposium on the Definition and Management of Anaphylaxis lists the following clinical criteria for diagnosis of anaphylaxis:

1. Acute onset of an illness (minutes to several hours) with involvement of the skin, mucosal tissue, or both (eg, generalized hives; pruritus or flushing; swollen lips, tongue, uvula)
   And at least 1 of the following:
   a. Respiratory compromise (eg, dyspnea, wheeze-bronchospasm, stridor, reduced peak expiratory flow, hypoxemia)

Table 6
Severity of asthma exacerbation assessment

Symptoms	Mild	Moderate	Severe	Near Death
Breathless	While walking	While talking	At rest	Decreased effort
Speaking	In sentences	In phrases	In words	Unable
Alertness	May be agitated	Usually agitated	Usually agitated	Confused
Respiratory Rate (breaths/min)	Increased	Increased	>30	>30, imminent failure
Accessory Muscle Use	Usually not	Commonly	Usually	Usually
Wheeze	Moderate	Loud	Loud or silent	Silent
Heart Rate (beats/min)	<100	100–120	>120	±
Saturation (%)	>95	92–94	<90	<90

    b. Reduced blood pressure (BP) or associated symptoms of end-organ dysfunction (eg, hypotonia [collapse], syncope, incontinence)

2. Two or more of the following that occur rapidly after exposure to a likely allergen for that patient:
    a. Involvement of the skin-mucosal tissue
    b. Respiratory compromise
    c. Reduced BP or associated symptoms
    d. Persistent gastrointestinal symptoms (eg, crampy abdominal pain, vomiting)

3. Reduced BP after exposure to known allergen for that patient:
    a. Infants and children: low systolic BP (age specific) or greater than 30% decrease in systolic BP
    b. Adults: systolic BP of less than 90 mm Hg or greater than 30% decrease from that person's baseline

It is the respiratory compromise that is relevant to this article, and it is important to recognize that treating the allergic component of these symptoms is necessary to save the patients.

Parenchymal Dyspnea

Now EMS is at the back door with a 60-year-old patient with a history of COPD and congestive heart failure (CHF). He is in respiratory distress with audible wheezing and tripoding. He is diaphoretic, hypertensive, and has pitting edema to his knees. They have given albuterol with no improvement of his symptoms.

Acute dyspnea is the most common symptom of patients presenting with heart failure.[17] Eighty percent of patients with acutely decompensated heart failure present through the ED with a chief complaint of dyspnea.[18] This symptom is related to both pulmonary and systemic fluid overload and also low cardiac output. American College of Emergency Physicians clinical policy makes level B recommendations that standard clinical judgment can be improved with the use of a single B-type natriuretic peptide (BNP) or N-terminal pro–B-type natriuretic peptide measurement to rule in or out the diagnosis of CHF.[19] However, the true utility, may be in patients with dyspnea not expected to have a CHF exacerbation, when finding a positive BNP would change management and allow a faster initiation of treatment.[20]

Carpenter and colleagues[20] found that the classic constellation of symptoms (jugular venous distension, peripheral edema, rales, and S3) were no more predictive of patients with both pulmonary edema on chest radiograph and an increased BNP level greater than 500 pg/dL than any individual finding alone. Although rales were the most sensitive finding tested for either outcome, they had specificity of only about 50% each. Jugular venous distention and S3 gallop were the individual findings most predictive for pulmonary edema on radiograph or increased BNP level. Ultrasonography measurements of the inferior vena cava also improve diagnostic accuracy versus BNP and chest radiograph alone.[21]

The medics are back in your department, this time with a 75-year-old man with cough and fever. His family is worried that he has been eating less and is sleepier than at hospital discharge last week. In pneumonia, the diffusion of oxygen is limited by alveolar infiltrates, leading to shortness of breath. Common complaints and findings in community-acquired pneumonia include fever, cough, pleuritic chest pain, and sputum production, along with dyspnea. However, these clinical criteria may have a sensitivity as low as 50% compared with a chest radiograph.[22] On examination, many patients have crackles or evidence of consolidation. Guidelines from the Infectious Diseases Society of America and the American Thoracic Society, recommend chest radiograph in patients with suspected pneumonia, which may show lobular consolidation, interstitial infiltrate, or cavitation.[23] Although infiltrate with suggestive symptoms makes the diagnosis, infiltrate may not be visible initially on patients with volume depletion. It is appropriate to treat empirically for 24 to 48 hours in these cases and to reimage when hydration is restored.

The management of pneumonia requires history to allow classification based on the setting in which the illness was acquired. The Infectious Disease Society of America and American Thoracic Society define the types of pneumonia as follows:[24] Hospital-acquired pneumonia (HAP) is "pneumonia that occurs 48 hours or more after admission which was not incubating at the time of admission." Ventilator-associated pneumonia (VAP) arises "more than 48-72 hours after endotracheal intubation." In addition, health care–associated pneumonia (HCAP) is diagnosed in any patient who is "hospitalized in an acute care hospital for two or more days within 90 days of the infection, resided in a nursing home or long-term care facility, received recent IV antibiotic therapy, chemotherapy or wound care within the past 30 days of the current infection or attended a hospital or hemodialysis clinic." Community-acquired pneumonia is not acquired in any of these situations. These classifications identify typical pathogens and guide appropriate initial management. Important historical exposures and risk factors to refine treatment are summarized in **Table 7**.[23]

The American Thoracic Society along with the Infectious Disease Society of America's consensus statement offers 4 important principles in the initial management and evaluation of adult patients with bacterial HAP, VAP, or HCAP; the most important to be accomplished in the ED is to promptly treat with "appropriate and adequate therapy" to decrease mortality.[24]

Circulatory Dyspnea

After a brief delay, you see a 28-year-old woman with shortness of breath and chest pain. She smokes, uses hormonal birth control, and reports that her symptoms started when she came back from a business trip. Pulmonary embolism (PE) interferes with both ventilation and perfusion. It ultimately causes circulatory collapse because of obstruction of right ventricular outflow eventually causing increased pulmonary artery pressure and failure of the right then left ventricles. Before circulatory collapse, echocardiography can show signs of right ventricular (RV) strain, including dilatation of the right ventricle, RV hypokinesis, paradoxic septal wall motion, McConnell sign (hypokinesis of the free RV wall with sparing of the apex), and tricuspid regurgitation.[25]

Dresden and colleagues[26] supported the use of ultrasonography in moderate-risk to high-risk patients to determine whether the patients were appropriate for anticoagulation while awaiting definitive imaging. Early anticoagulation is recommended to improve mortality and there is evidence to support anticoagulation before diagnosis in patients with a Wells score greater than 4 who will have a delay to diagnosis of more than 1 hour and 40 minutes.[27,28]

The assessment of patients with dyspnea and concern for PE requires a series of risk stratification. One common method is to use Wells criteria[29] (**Box 1**) in patients with suspicion for PE; although other stratification tools exist, none has been shown to be clearly superior. When there is low clinical suspicion for PE, PERC (pulmonary embolism rule-out criteria)[30] rules or D-dimer testing may be applied.[27] If PERC (**Box 2**) is negative, or there is intermediate pretest probability for PE with negative high-sensitivity D-dimer, no further testing for PE is required.[27] When further testing is needed (positive D-dimer or high-sensitivity D-dimer not available), negative CT angiogram or low-probability VQ scan may be used to rule out PE.

Table 7
Common pathogens in community-acquired pneumonia

Condition	Commonly Encountered Pathogens
Alcoholism	*Streptococcus pneumoniae*, oral anaerobes, *Klebsiella pneumoniae*, *Acinetobacter* species, *Mycobacterium tuberculosis*
COPD and/or smoking	*Haemophilus influenzae*, *Pseudomonas aeruginosa*, *Legionella* species, *S pneumonia*, *Moraxella catarrhalis*, *Chlamydophila pneumoniae*
Aspiration	Gram-negative enteric pathogens, oral anaerobes
Lung abscess	CA-MRSA, oral anaerobes, endemic fungal pneumonia, *M tuberculosis*, atypical mycobacteria
Exposure to bat or bird droppings	*Histoplasma capsulatum*
Exposure to birds	*Chlamydophila psittaci* (if poultry: avian influenza)
Exposure to rabbits	*Francisella tularensis*
Exposure to farm animals or parturient cats	*Coxiella burnetii* (Q fever)
HIV infection (early)	*S pneumoniae, H influenzae, M tuberculosis*
HIV infection (late)	The pathogens listed for early infection plus *Pneumocystis jirovecii, Cryptococcus, Histoplasma, Aspergillus*, atypical mycobacteria (especially *Mycobacterium kansasii*), *P aeruginosa, H influenzae*
Hotel or cruise ship stay in previous 2 wk	*Legionella* species
Travel to or residence in southwestern United States	*Coccidioides* species, Hantavirus
Travel to or residence in southeast and east Asia	*Burkholderia pseudomallei*, avian influenza, SARS
Influenza active in community	Influenza, *S pneumoniae, Staphylococcus aureus, H influenzae*
Cough>2 wk with whoop or post-tussive vomiting	*Bordetella pertussis*
Structural lung disease (eg, bronchiectasis)	*P aeruginosa, Burkholderia cepacia, S aureus*
Injection drug use	*S aureus*, anaerobes, *M tuberculosis, S pneumoniae*
Endobronchial obstruction	Anaerobes, *S pneumonia, H influenzae, S aureus*
In context of bioterrorism	*Bacillus anthracis* (anthrax), *Yersinia pestis* (plague), *Francisella tularensis* (tularemia)

Abbreviations: CA-MRSA, community-acquired methicillin-resistant *Staphylococcus aureus*; HIV, human immunodeficiency virus; SARS, severe acute respiratory syndrome.

From Mandell LA, Wunderink RG, Anzueto A, et al. Infectious Diseases Society of America/American Thoracic Society consensus guidelines on the management of community-acquired pneumonia in adults. Clin Infect Dis 2007;44(Suppl 2):S46; with permission.

In the next bed is a middle-aged woman with diabetes complaining of shortness of breath today. It was associated with some vague nausea and she says that she just does not feel good. Angina pectoris is cardiac chest pain in which oxygen demand outweighs myocardial oxygen supply; in this case caused by occlusion of coronary arteries. Although typically chest pain is a part of the presentation, dyspnea alone may be the initial complaint, termed an anginal equivalent. In one recent large series of patients undergoing stress testing, patients with dyspnea alone were at increased

---

Box 1
Wells criteria for pulmonary embolism

- Clinical signs and symptoms of deep vein thrombosis (DVT): +3
- PE is the main diagnosis or equally likely: +3
- Heart Rate greater than 100 beats/min: +1.5
- Immobilization >3 days or surgery in last 4 weeks: +1.5
- History of prior PE/deep venous thrombosis (DVT): +1.5
- Hemoptysis: +1
- Malignancy with treatment within 6 months or palliative: +1

Less than or equal to 1.5 = low risk, 1.3% chance of PE in ED population; 2 to 6 = moderate risk, 16.2% chance of PE in ED population; greater than 6 = high risk, 40.6% chance of PE in ED population
    Adapted from Wells PS, Anderson DR, Rodger M, et al. Excluding pulmonary embolism at the bedside without diagnostic imaging: Management of patients with suspected pulmonary embolism presenting to the emergency department by using a simple clinical model and D-dimer. Ann Intern Med 2001;135:99.

---

risk of death from cardiac causes. Patients asked simply whether they experienced shortness of breath were considered dyspneic. The subset with no prior known coronary artery disease had more than 4 times the risk of sudden cardiac death versus asymptomatic patients and more than twice the risk of those with typical angina.[31] Clinicians should consider past medical history and risk factors when assessing dyspnea for cardiac causes such as acute myocardial infarction and acute coronary syndrome. Appropriate testing includes bedside electrocardiogram, troponin, and chest radiograph.

The department eventually settles down and you are able to do some charting until a young man comes in with visible respiratory distress. He is tall and thin, smokes regularly, and reports sudden onset of severely painful breathing. Pneumothorax occurs when air enters the plural space between the chest wall and the lung. Typically only a thin serous layer exists between the visceral and parietal pleura. Air enters this potential space only when there is damage to the lung or chest wall, or a gas-producing pleural space infection. The classic risk factors for bleb rupture causing spontaneous

---

Box 2
Pulmonary embolism rule-out criteria

- Further work-up recommended if any of the following are present:
    - Age greater than or equal to 50 years
    - Pulse greater than or equal to 100 beats/min
    - Oxygen saturation less than 95%
    - Hemoptysis
    - Unilateral leg swelling
    - History of PE/DVT
    - Exogenous estrogen use
    - Surgery or trauma within 4 weeks that required hospitalization or intubation
- If none are present, probability of PE is less than 2%.

Adapted from Kline JA, Courtney DM, Babrhel C, et al. Prospective multicenter evaluation of the pulmonary embolism rule-out criteria. J Thromb Haemost 2008;6(5):773.

pneumothorax are tall men, although smoking has been suggested to increase the risk of rupture by damaging the pleural layer.

Pneumothoraces may be identified by ultrasonography, chest radiograph, or CT. Treatment may be guided by cause, severity, comorbidities, interventions such as positive pressure ventilation, size of the pneumothorax, and patient's preference. Recent studies suggest that uncomplicated spontaneous pneumothorax in patients not undergoing positive pressure ventilation may be treated as successfully with needle aspiration as with other more invasive chest drains, regardless of size.[32]

Tension pneumothorax is a serious event requiring immediate needle decompression to avert loss of cardiac output and arrest. However, recent review shows that the classic presentation of tension pneumothorax with hypotension, absent breath sounds, and deviated trachea may not be immediately seen in patients with spontaneous, unassisted respiration.[33] Because of the slower development of the accumulation of air and pressure variations, spontaneously breathing patients may compensate much longer and present atypically, as shown in **Table 8**. Thus, clinicians must remain vigilant.

Compensatory Dyspnea

This article focuses on the cardiopulmonary system as the source of the problem in acutely dyspneic patients. It is important to also consider that the appearance of shortness of breath, tachypnea, or other typical symptoms of dyspnea may result from changing metabolic demands. These patients may appear, on the surface, to be in respiratory distress; they may be tachypneic, tachycardic, even pale or diaphoretic. In these cases, the clinician's responsibility is to identify and fix the true problem in order to improve the respiratory symptoms.

Severely anemic patients have limited oxygen carrying capacity. Their bodies therefore experience oxygen hunger, which can manifest as shortness of breath. Patients with dysfunctional hemoglobins secondary to irreversibly bound atoms or toxins may also be functionally anemic with the same symptoms.

People's bodies attempt at all costs to maintain equilibrium. Therefore, in metabolic acidoses (such as diabetic ketoacidosis), chemoreceptors detect acidosis and

Table 8
Findings in tension pneumothorax

Unassisted Ventilation	Positive Pressure Ventilation
Spontaneous respiration with air passing through 1-way flap	Assisted ventilation forces air through pleural defect into pleural space
Compensatory mechanisms delay collapse: • Tachycardia and accessory muscle use caused by tachypnea, increased tidal volume, and negative movement of the opposite side of the chest • BP is maintained because of limits in the pressure of the pneumothorax on mediastinum and hemithorax	Sudden hemodynamic and respiratory compromise: • Sedation may increase inspiratory pressure • Intrapleural pressure is increased throughout respiratory cycle
Venous siphon resulting from negative intrathoracic pressure in the opposite side of the chest returns blood to the heart	Decreased venous return leads to hypotension and cardiac arrest

Adapted from Roberts DJ, Leigh-smith S, Faris PD, et al. Clinical presentation of patients with tension pneumothorax: a systematic review. Ann Surg 2015;261(6):1069.

stimulate the respiratory center to hyperventilate. Both the rate and the depth of venti-lation often increase, leading to both tachypnea and hyperpnea, at times referred to as Kussmaul respirations. This compensatory response is crucial for survival and should not be mistaken for dyspnea. It is equally important to realize that an increase in alve-olar ventilation is not always a compensatory response (to acidosis or to primary pul-monary disorders) and hypocapnia may cause primary respiratory alkalosis, from central nervous system compromise, toxins (eg, salicylates), anxiety, or pain.[34] In these patients, imaging rarely reveals a source of dyspnea, but clinical suspicion based on history and examination, including signs such as the fruity breath of ketone-mia, the pallor of anemia, or the cyanosis of toxic hemoglobinopathies, directs pro-viders toward appropriate laboratory testing and treatment.

Diagnosis of Exclusion

In addition, sometimes dyspnea is not dyspnea. Acute anxiety and panic disorder can present as shortness of breath, tachypnea, or hyperventilation. Patients with panic disorder often describe symptoms similar to those of patients with true airway obstruction despite their normal pulmonary function. It has been suggested that these patients have abnormal proprioception, experiencing dyspnea without abnormal stim-uli.[35] However, patients with a history of pulmonary disease can also have pure panic episodes. Arterial blood gas may be useful in diagnosing anxiety-related hyperventilation.[36]

Severe pain can also induce abnormal respiratory patterns. Like compensatory problems, pain and anxiety can be managed by managing their causes. Treat pain. Reduce stress and anxiety with words, behaviors, or, if necessary, medications. How-ever, air hunger and difficulty breathing also make individuals anxious. Be sure to avoid premature diagnosis of a purely anxiety-based concern without first evaluating for more dangerous disorders.

SUMMARY

Acute dyspnea presents commonly to the ED and it is imperative that emergency phy-sicians be prepared to stabilize patients' oxygenation and ventilation, which requires careful and efficient consideration of the differential diagnosis. Using cues from the history and physical examination, practitioners may guide the work-up and treatment to identify a parenchymal, obstructive, circulatory, or compensatory cause of dys-pnea. Early use of bedside testing, including ultrasonography, may limit unnecessary tests and save time in determining the best treatment course. Thus ensuring both the best care for the patient and also the physician's ability to readily respond to the next case.

REFERENCES

1. Prekker ME, Feemster LC, Hough CL, et al. The epidemiology and outcome of prehospital respiratory distress. Acad Emerg Med 2014;21(5):543–50.
2. American Thoracic Society. Dyspnea. Mechanisms, assessment, and manage-ment: a consensus statement. Am J Respir Crit Care Med 1999;159:321–40.
3. Schwartzstein RM, Lewis A. Chapter 29: Dyspnea. In: Broaddus V, Mason RC, Ernst JD, et al, editors. Murray & Nadel's textbook of respiratory medicine. 6th edition. Philadelphia: Elsevier Health Sciences, Saunders/Elsevier; 2015. p. 490–1.
4. Kajimoto K, Madeen K, Nakayama T, et al. Rapid evaluation by lung-cardiac infe-rior vena cava (LCI) integrated ultrasound for differentiating heart failure from

pulmonary disease as the cause of acute dyspnea in the emergency setting. Cardiovasc Ultrasound 2012;10:49.

5. Anderson KL, Jenq KY, Fields JM, et al. Diagnosing heart failure among acutely dyspneic patients with cardiac, inferior vena cava and lung ultrasonography. Am J Emerg Med 2013;31:1208–14.

6. Russell FM, Ehrman RR, Cosby K, et al. Diagnosing acute heart failure in patients with undifferentiated dyspnea: a lung and cardiac ultrasound (LuCUS) protocol. Acad Emerg Med 2015;22(2):182–91.

7. Feng LB, Pines JM, Yusuf HR, et al. U.S. trends in computed tomography use and diagnoses in emergency department visits by patients with symptoms suggestive of pulmonary embolism, 2001-2009. Acad Emerg Med 2013;20(10):1033–40.

8. Huckins DS, Price LL, Gilley K. Utilization and yield of chest computed tomographic angiography associated with low positive D-dimer levels. J Emerg Med 2012;43:211–20.

9. Qaseem A, Alguire P, Dall P, et al. Appropriate use of screening and diagnostic tests to foster, high-value, cost-conscious care. Ann Intern Med 2012;156:147–9.

10. Coco AS, O'gurek DT. Increased emergency department computed tomography use for common chest symptoms without clear patient benefits. J Am Board Fam Med 2012;25(1):33–41.

11. Chapter 8, The thorax and lungs. In: Bickley LS, Szilagyi PG, editors. Bates' guide to physical examination and history taking. 11th edition. Philadelphia: Lippincott Williams & Wilkins; 2013. p. 301.

12. Global Initiative for Asthma. Diagnosis of diseases of chronic airflow limitation: asthma, COPD and asthma-COPD overlap syndrome (ACOS). 2015. Available at: http://www.ginasthma.org/documents/14/Asthma%2C-COPD-and-Asthma-COPD-Overlap-Syndrome-%28ACOS%29. Accessed May 1, 2015.

13. Husain AN. Chapter 15, The lung. In: Kumar V, Abbas AK, Aster JC, editors. Robbins and Cotran pathologic basis of disease. 9th edition. Philadelphia: WB Saunders; 2014. p. 679.

14. Ram FS, Rodriguez-Roison R, Granados-Navarrete A, et al. Antibiotics for exacerbations of chronic obstructive pulmonary disease. Cochrane Database Syst Rev 2006;(2):CD004403.

15. Sampson HA, Munoz-Furlong A, Campbell RL, et al. Second Symposium on the Definition and Management of Anaphylaxis: summary Report – Second National Institute of Allergy and Immunology. Ann Emerg Med 2006;47(4):373–80.

16. Simons FES, Ardusso LRF, Dimov V, et al. World Allergy Organization anaphylaxis guidelines: 2013 update of the evidence base. Int Arch Allergy Immunol 2013; 162:193–204.

17. Pang PS, Collins SP, Sauser K, et al. Assessment of dyspnea early in acute heart failure: patient characteristics and response differences between Likert and visual analog scales. Acad Emerg Med 2014;21(6):659–66.

18. Fonarow GC. The Acute Decompensated Heart Failure National Registry (ADHERE): opportunities to improve care of patients hospitalized with acute decompensated heart failure. Rev Cardiovasc Med 2003;4(Suppl 7):S21–30.

19. Silvers SM, Howell JM, Kosowsky JM, et al. Clinical policy: critical issues in the evaluation and management of adult patients presenting to the emergency department with acute heart failure syndromes. Ann Emerg Med 2007;49(5): 627–69.

20. Carpenter CR, Keim SM, Worster A, et al. Brain natriuretic peptide in the evaluation of emergency department dyspnea: is there a role? J Emerg Med 2012;42(2): 197–205.

21. Miller JB, Sen A, Strote SR, et al. Inferior vena cava assessment in the bedside diagnosis of acute heart failure. Am J Emerg Med 2012;30(5):778–83.
22. Metlay JP, Fine MJ. Testing strategies in the initial management of patients with community-acquired pneumonia. Ann Intern Med 2003;138:109.
23. Mandell LA, Wunderink RG, Anzueto A, et al. Infectious Diseases Society of America/American Thoracic Society consensus guidelines on the management of community-acquired pneumonia in adults. Clin Infect Dis 2007;44(Suppl 2): S27–72.
24. American Thoracic Society, Infectious Diseases Society of America. Guidelines for the management of adults with hospital-acquired, ventilator-associated, and healthcare-associated pneumonia. Am J Respir Crit Care Med 2005;171(4): 388–416.
25. Kucher N, Rossi E, DeRosa M, et al. Prognostic role of echocardiography among patients with acute pulmonary embolism and a systolic arterial pressure of 90 mm Hg or higher. Arch Intern Med 2005;165:1777–81.
26. Dresden S, Mitchell P, Rahimi L, et al. Right ventricular dilatation on bedside echocardiography performed by emergency physicians aids in the diagnosis of pulmonary embolism. Ann Emerg Med 2014;63(1):16–24.
27. Fesmire FM, Brown MD, Espinosa JA, et al. Critical issues in the evaluation and management of adult patients presenting to the emergency department with suspected pulmonary embolism. Ann Emerg Med 2011;57(6):628–52.e75.
28. Blondon M, Righini M, Aujesky D, et al. Usefulness of preemptive anticoagulation in patients with suspected pulmonary embolism: a decision analysis. Chest 2012; 142:697–703.
29. Wells PS, Anderson DR, Rodger M, et al. Excluding pulmonary embolism at the bedside without diagnostic imaging: management of patients with suspected pulmonary embolism presenting to the emergency department by using a simple clinical model and D-dimer. Ann Intern Med 2001;135:98–107.
30. Kline JA, Courtney DM, Babrhel C, et al. Prospective multicenter evaluation of the pulmonary embolism rule-out criteria. J Thromb Haemost 2008;6(5):772–80.
31. Abidov A, Rozanski A, Hachamovitch R, et al. Prognostic significance of dyspnea in patients referred for cardiac stress testing. N Engl J Med 2005;353(18): 1889–98.
32. Zehtabchi S, Rios CL. Management of emergency department patients with primary spontaneous pneumothorax: needle aspiration or tube thoracostomy? Ann Emerg Med 2008;51(1):91–100, 100.e1.
33. Roberts DJ, Leigh-smith S, Faris PD, et al. Clinical presentation of patients with tension pneumothorax: a systematic review. Ann Surg 2015;261:1068–78.
34. Morris CG, Low J. Metabolic acidosis in the critically ill: part 1. Classification and pathophysiology. Anaesthesia 2008;63(3):294–301.
35. Smoller JW, Pollack MH, Otto MW, et al. Panic anxiety, dyspnea, and respiratory disease. Am J Respir Crit Care Med 1996;154:6–17.
36. Burri E, Potocki M, Drexler B, et al. Value of arterial blood gas analysis in patients with acute dyspnea: an observational study. Crit Care 2011;15(3):R145.
37. Syrjala H, Broas M, Suramo I, et al. High resolution computed tomography for the diagnosis of community-acquired pneumonia. Clin Infect Dis 1998;27:358–63.

Advances in Point-of-Care Thoracic Ultrasound

Zareth Irwin, MD*, Justin O. Cook, MD

KEYWORDS

- Pulmonary ultrasound • Pneumothorax • Pulmonary edema • Pleural effusion
- Hemothorax • Pneumonia

KEY POINTS

- Pulmonary ultrasound allows for rapid diagnosis of pneumothorax, pulmonary edema, pneumonia, and intrathoracic free fluid.
- Pulmonary ultrasound is more sensitive and specific than chest radiograph for many pulmonary conditions.
- Pulmonary ultrasound is the most rapidly advancing form of pulmonary imaging.

 Videos of various normal and abnormal lung ultrasound findings accompany this article at http://www.emed.theclinics.com/

Although technological advances continue to improve the imaging quality and diagnostic capabilities of computed tomography (CT) scanning, chest radiography remains the mainstay of pulmonary diagnostic imaging in emergent settings because of its relative portability and ease of acquisition and image interpretation. However, compared with pulmonary ultrasound, which has seen rapid growth in the past decade, radiography has inherent limitations.

First, although chest x-ray is portable, it requires a technologist, a machine that is typically not located in patients' rooms, and often requires development in an area remote from patients. The machine itself is large, and the process of obtaining the image requires moving patients to some degree regardless of the type of study. These factors are insignificant at times; but in the setting of a critically ill patient when real estate in the resuscitation bay is limited and time-sensitive interventions are necessary, radiography can be disruptive to patient care. Additionally, although minimal, the ionizing radiation associated with radiography is not insignificant,

The authors have nothing to disclose.
Northwest Acute Care Specialists, Emergency medicine, 825 Northeast Multnomah St, Portland, OR 97232, USA
* Corresponding author. 4826 Northeast Alameda, Portland, OR 97213.
E-mail address: zarethirwin@mac.com

Emerg Med Clin N Am 34 (2016) 151–157
http://dx.doi.org/10.1016/j.emc.2015.09.003
0733-8627/16/$ – see front matter © 2016 Elsevier Inc. All rights reserved.

especially as radiographs are repeated to monitor patients' condition and response to treatment.

Perhaps more importantly is the fact that chest radiography is relatively insensitive for findings such as pleural fluid and pneumothorax, especially in supine patients.[1–3] These limitations, in conjunction with advances in ultrasound technology and more widespread training have led to increased use of this technology for the evaluation of pathologic conditions in emergent settings.

Ultrasound machines have become more portable, with decreased boot-up time, while simultaneously providing improved image quality and ease of image acquisition. These factors make thoracic ultrasound ideal for emergency departments, operating rooms, intensive care units, and the prehospital setting. Bedside ultrasound has been a core competency of American Board of Emergency Medicine–accredited emergency medicine training programs since 2008, and most medical schools now have extensive ultrasound education integrated into their curriculum.

Although user dependent, in the right hands, ultrasound is more sensitive than chest radiographs for many types of pulmonary pathology[1–3] and approaches sensitivities and specificities of CT for pneumonia.[4–6] Additionally, it is easily done at the bedside without patient care interruption and can be used in real time to guide procedures (eg, reduction of pneumothorax). Serial ultrasounds are ideal for monitoring changes in patients' condition and response to treatment, as there is minimal lag between physiologic changes and imaging findings. For these reasons, pulmonary ultrasound has high-yield applications in critically ill and injured patients.

Among imaging modalities for respiratory emergencies, pulmonary ultrasound has seen the greatest recent advancement. This article reviews the advantages of pulmonary ultrasound and demonstrates imaging technique as well as ultrasound findings of normal lung and common pathologic states.

BASIC THORACIC EXAMINATION

The initial goal of thoracic ultrasound in dyspneic patients should focus on detecting changes at the lung periphery. Evaluation for the presence or absence of movement between the visceral and parietal pleura (lung sliding; Videos 1 and 2) will assess for pneumothorax. Imaging of the costophrenic angles should be performed to detect pleural fluid, as in the setting of an effusion or hemothorax (Video 3). Parenchymal processes, such as pneumonia and pulmonary edema or contusion, are readily identified by bedside ultrasound via utilization of greater depth of field.

Pneumothorax

The initial diagnosis of pneumothorax has classically been via chest radiograph, but this modality is insensitive for small pneumothoraces (especially in supine patients). The sensitivity of bedside ultrasound for the detection of pneumothorax exceeds that of standard chest radiographs, with sensitivity approaching that of CT.[1,2,4] Radiographic imaging remains the easiest means for rapidly estimating pneumothorax size, but ultrasound can also be used to determine the extent of pneumothorax by mapping out areas where there is an absence of lung sliding.

Technique

During a focused examination for pneumothorax, a linear transducer is optimal because of its ability to provide high-resolution images at shallow depths. However, lower-frequency microconvex, phased array, or curved transducers can also be used. Lower frequency probes offer the advantage of deeper penetration into the lung parenchyma, which may reveal additional pathology.

With the probe marker cephalad, orient the linear transducer longitudinally. Beginning at the second or third intercostal space, visualize the bright, hyperechoic pleura between the ribs (the ribs appear as bright, semicircular surfaces with distal shadows); this has been referred to as the bat-wing sign (**Fig. 1**). Staying paramedian, image the pleural interface in at least 3 different interspaces, always comparing bilaterally, with attention focused on the most likely location for pneumothorax (ie, the least-dependent area of the chest, the area to which air would be expected to track). Depending on the clinical situation, this examination may be performed as part of more comprehensive lung protocols, which generally use a curved or phased-array transducer.

Normal lung is composed of little mass and abundant air, which deflects and scatters echoes to the detriment of obtaining distinct deep images. This composition changes for diseased lung. In either case, the pleural interface is easily appreciated as a bright (hyperechoic) line between darker rib shadows. Once the pleura has been identified, lung sliding is appreciated as the visceral pleura slides back and forth against the stationary parietal pleural with respiration. In the absence of pneumothorax, comet tail artifacts may also be seen at the pleural interface (see Video 1). These artifacts, which appear as bright beads with hyperechoic tails projecting distally, are a normal finding resulting from microbubbles existing between the pleural layers. Additionally, A lines, a type of artifact that results in recurring, horizontal, hyperechoic lines occurring at regular intervals from the pleural line, represent normal, aerated lung parenchyma (Video 4).

The absence of lung sliding is highly sensitive but not specific for pneumothorax. As lung sliding represents movement between the layers of the pleura, other causes for lack of lung sliding, such as mainstem intubation on the contralateral side, previous pleurodesis, severe pneumonia, and acute respirator distress syndrome (ARDS), do exist[7,8] (see Video 2).

When the subtle movement of lung sliding is difficult to discern, movement mode (M mode) may increase the sensitivity of this finding. In M mode, data from a single vertical slice of the image (usually displayed as a vertical green line on first press of the M mode button) are displayed over time. With M mode, normal lung sliding will produce a

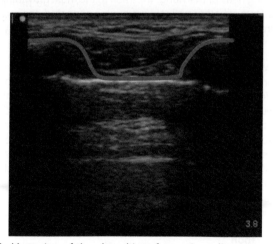

Fig. 1. The so-called bat wing of the pleural interface, using a linear transducer. The wings of the bat (*pink line*) overlie the superficial aspect of ribs, which cause shadowing far afield. The body of the bat is the brightly hyperechoic or white pleural line.

beach or seashore sign. This sign is demonstrated by the presence of horizontal lines (waves) above the pleural line and a granular appearance (sand) deep to the pleural line (Video 5). In the setting of pneumothorax, there is no pleural interface for sliding to occur. This lack of lung sliding is demonstrated on M mode by loss of the beach, resulting in the presence of linear lines above and below the level of the parietal pleura. This sign is often referred to as the stratosphere or barcode sign (Video 6).

Imaging both sides of the chest will help increase sensitivity and allow for comparison to help discern between normal and vaguely abnormal findings. As the absence of sliding will only be evident in the interspaces where the pneumothorax is located, detection of very small pneumothoraces, or those in locations difficult to image (apical, paramediastinal), can be challenging. Despite this, the sensitivity of ultrasound for the detection of pneumothorax approaches 90%, with a positive likelihood ratio of 50 and negative likelihood ratio of 0.09.[9]

An additional sign, the lung pulse, suggests the direct apposition of parietal and visceral pleura (ie, absence of pneumothorax). This finding can be particularly useful when assessing areas of lung that, by virtue of its close proximity to the heart, may not otherwise clearly demonstrate an appearance of lung sliding.[10] The lung pulse appears as a pulsatile movement of the visceral on the parietal pleura, at the same frequency as the heart rate. The presence of the lung pulse excludes pneumothorax in that area.

The presence of lung sliding, A lines, and the lung pulse are all findings that exclude pneumothorax; but their absence is not specific for the presence of pneumothorax. However, if present, the lung point is very specific for pneumothorax (reported specificity of 100%)[11] (Video 7). The lung point is the interface between the presence and absence of lung sliding in a single rib interspace. It is the visualization of the exact point where the separation between the layers of pleura begins. The visualization of lung points rules in pneumothorax, and determining their location allows estimation of pneumothorax size.

Pleural Effusion

As fluid is a good conductor of sound, ultrasound is very sensitive for free fluid in the chest. Unlike free air in the chest, which will track to the most gravitationally independent area, fluid, being heavier than lung, will track to the most gravitationally dependent area in the chest. Thus, whether patients are supine or seated, the most sensitive area for detection of free fluid will be just above the diaphragm posteriorly and laterally.

Technique

Use a probe that will allow for a relatively deep imaging field (eg, phased array or curvilinear). With the probe marker cephalad, place the transducer in the midaxillary to posterior axillary line (depends on patient position) within the 8th to 11th interspaces. Fresh blood or pleural fluid will appear black (anechoic) or with some internal echoes if partly clotted (hypoechoic) between the hyperechoic diaphragm and pleural surface of the lung, which can sometimes be seen floating in this fluid collection. The pleural interface can be rapidly assessed for an intrathoracic collection of fluid, such as hemothorax or pleural effusion (Video 8). These views are often obtained in the right upper quadrant and left upper quadrant views of the FAST examination, with the transducer angled more cephalad, or with patients seated upright and leaning forward when evaluating for a medical effusion.

Parenchymal Evaluation

Beyond detection of pneumothorax and pleural effusion, a more comprehensive lung examination allows for elucidation of many other disease processes in the lung. The optimal low-frequency transducer for a comprehensive lung examination is debatable; microconvex and convex transducers provide high image quality, but phased-array probes offer the convenience of performing concomitant cardiac imaging or FAST scans without changing the transducer. Although the overall clinical data do not differ significantly between transducers, the machine should be set to perform a minimum amount of signal processing.[8] This setting will allow for enhanced visualization of artifacts (eg, A lines, B lines, comet tails), which is crucial for optimal lung imaging.

Protocols for comprehensive lung examinations exist and may be helpful to ensure that a complete examination is performed. One such protocol divides each anterior lung into 4 zones, with the anterior axillary line forming the vertical line bisecting this zone, the horizontal line at about the level of the nipple, bound anteriorly by parasternal line and posteriorly by the posterior axillary line; such a 4-zone-per-side approach allows for a rapid yet systematic lung evaluation.[12]

Lung Interstitial Syndrome

Interstitial fluid is readily identified by the presence and density of B lines. These vertical reverberation artifacts are thought to be formed by an acoustic mismatch between the lung and the surrounding tissues, such that the ultrasound beam is partly reflected as the beam travels farther afield.[8]

B lines (Video 9) are laserlike and appear as discrete, vertical, hyperechoic artifacts that move with respiration, obliterate A lines, and extend brightly, without diminution, from the pleural interface to the far field of the image (as distinct from normal comet tails of lung sliding, which trail off only after a few centimeters as they project far field).[10] Although the presence of scattered B lines at the lung bases can be normal, the presence of 3 or more B lines in a longitudinal plane in any single rib interspace indicates increased interstitial fluid.[10]

The specific distribution of B lines and the appearance of the pleural interface can help elucidate the cause of the increased interstitial fluid.[8] As one might expect, B lines caused by cardiogenic pulmonary edema tend to be bilateral, gravitationally dependent, and symmetric. Acute lung injury or ARDS will have a more irregular, patchy pattern of bilateral B lines, often with adjacent subpleural consolidations and fragmentation of the pleural interface. Point-of-care echocardiogram with or without ultrasound of the inferior vena cava can further assist in determining the cause of interstitial fluid. Overall, the accuracy of point-of-care ultrasound for the detection of cardiogenic pulmonary edema is high (94% sensitivity, 92% specificity).[13]

Lung Consolidation and Severe Contusion

Although healthy lung parenchyma consists primarily of air, and thus provides little meaningful sonographic information, in the setting of infection, the interstitial space consolidates and allows for sound transmission. In this case, the lung appears more like a solid organ and takes on the appearance of liver (termed hepatization) (Video 10). This finding is well correlated with findings of consolidation on chest radiograph and CT. Lung ultrasound for pneumonia may be superior to chest radiograph, with sensitivities and specificities approaching that of CT, for both hospitalized and emergency department patients.[14,15]

The appearance of consolidated lung can be seen in the setting of pneumonia, focal pulmonary contusion, focal infarct, and atelectasis, with the most common causes being pneumonia and atelectasis. Lung ultrasound helps distinguish between consolidation and atelectasis (which can be difficult with chest radiograph), as consolidation leaves the bronchi unobstructed and air moving within the consolidation will generate air bronchograms. In contrast, atelectasis causes bronchial plugging, and the air within the consolidation will be static.

Monitoring Pulmonary Function

Unlike other forms of pulmonary imaging, ultrasound demonstrates changes in clinical condition in real time. A decrease in the prevalence of B lines can be seen within 30 minutes of initiation of positive pressure ventilation in patients with pulmonary edema.[16,17] Similarly, fluid-overloaded patients undergoing dialysis show real-time resolution of B lines as their volume status improves.[18] This ability to closely follow the response to treatment allows for ongoing real-time treatment decisions.

SUMMARY

Point-of-care ultrasound is widely used for rapid diagnosis and treatment of many emergent conditions. Portable ultrasound machines are now commonplace in emergency departments, intensive care units, and operating rooms. Pulmonary ultrasound is highly accurate for the identification of pneumothorax, hemothorax, pleural effusions, infiltrates, and interstitial fluid. Additionally, it provides real-time information of treatment response. In the future, lung ultrasound will likely replace routine chest radiography.

SUPPLEMENTARY DATA

Supplementary data related to this article can be found online at http://dx.doi.org/10.1016/j.emc.2015.09.003.

REFERENCES

1. Rowan KR, Kirkpatrick AW, Liu D, et al. Traumatic pneumothorax detection with thoracic ultrasound; correlation with chest radiography and CT-initial experience. Radiology 2002;225:210–4.
2. Blaivas M, Lyon M, Duggal S. A prospective comparison of supine chest radiography and bedside ultrasound for the diagnosis of traumatic pneumothorax. Acad Emerg Med 2005;12:844–9.
3. Grimberg A, Shigueko DC, Atallah AN, et al. Diagnostic accuracy of sonography for pleural effusion: systematic review. Sao Paulo Med J 2010;128:90–5.
4. Cortellaro F, Colombo S, Coen D, et al. Pulmonary ultrasound is an accurate diagnostic tool for the diagnosis of pneumonia in the emergency department. Emerg Med J 2012;29(1):19–23.
5. Raja AS, Jacobus CH. Systematic review snapshot: how accurate is ultrasonography for the detection of pneumothorax? Ann Emerg Med 2013;61:207–8.
6. Lobo V, Weingrow D, Perera P, et al. Thoracic ultrasonography. Crit Care Clin 2014;20:93–117.
7. Lichtenstein DA, Menu Y. A bedside ultrasound sign ruling out pneumothorax in the critically ill: lung sliding. Chest 1995;108:1345–8.
8. Gargani L, Volpicelli G. How I do it: lung ultrasound. Cardiovasc Ultrasound 2014;12:25–35.
9. Wilkerson RG, Stone MB. Sensitivity of bedside ultrasound and supine anteroposterior chest radiographs for the identification of pneumothorax after blunt trauma. Acad Emerg Med 2010;17:11–7.
10. Volpicelli G, Elbarbary M, Blaivas M, et al. International evidence-based recommendations for point-of-care lung ultrasound. Intensive Care Med 2012;38:577–91.

11. Lichtenstein D, Meziere G, Biderman P, et al. The "lung point": an ultrasound sign specific to pneumothorax. Intensive Care Med 2000;26:1434–40.
12. Volpicelli G, Mussa A, Garofalo G, et al. Bedside lung ultrasound in the assessment of alveolar-interstitial syndrome. Am J Emerg Med 2006;24:689–96.
13. Al Deeb M, Barbic S, Featherstone R, et al. Point-of-care ultrasonography for the diagnosis of acute cardiogenic pulmonary edema in patients presenting with acute dyspnea: a systematic review and meta-analysis. Acad Emerg Med 2014;21(8):844–52.
14. Reissig A, Kroegel C. Sonographic diagnosis and follow-up of pneumonia: a prospective study. Respiration 2007;74(5):535–47.
15. Parlamento S, Copetti R, Di Bartolomeo S. Evaluation of lung ultrasound for the diagnosis of pneumonia in the ED. AM J Emerg Med 2009;27:379–84.
16. Liteplo AS, Murray AF, Kimberley HH, et al. Real-time resolution of sonographic B-lines in a patient with pulmonary edema on continuous positive airway pressure. Am J Emerg Med 2010;28:541.e5–8.
17. Bouhemad B, Brisson H, Le-Guen M, et al. Bedside ultrasound assessment of positive end-expiratory pressure-induced lung recruitment. Am J Respir Crit Care Med 2011;183(3):314–7.
18. Noble VE, Murray AF, Capp R, et al. Ultrasound assessment for extravascular lung water in patients undergoing hemodialysis. Time course for resolution. Chest 2009;135:1433–9.

Index

Note: Page numbers of article titles are in **boldface** type.

Emerg Med Clin N Am 34 (2016) 159–164
http://dx.doi.org/10.1016/S0733-8627(15)00103-0
0733-8627/16/$ – see front matter © 2016 Elsevier Inc. All rights reserved.

Moving?

Make sure your subscription moves with you!

To notify us of your new address, find your **Clinics Account Number** (located on your mailing label above your name), and contact customer service at:

Email: journalscustomerservice-usa@elsevier.com

800-654-2452 (subscribers in the U.S. & Canada)
314-447-8871 (subscribers outside of the U.S. & Canada)

Fax number: 314-447-8029

Elsevier Health Sciences Division
Subscription Customer Service
3251 Riverport Lane
Maryland Heights, MO 63043

*To ensure uninterrupted delivery of your subscription, please notify us at least 4 weeks in advance of move.

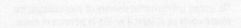

Printed and bound by CPI Group (UK) Ltd, Croydon, CR0 4YY

03/10/2024

01040486-0017